Where there is ecstasy, there is Creation;
Where there is no ecstasy, there is no Creation.
In the Infinite, there is ecstasy;
There is no ecstasy in the finite.
Chandogya Upanishad

IN ECSTASY THROUGH TANTRA, Dr. Jonn Mumford celebrates the joyous and mystical depths of sexual love. Over the past decade, we have become more free and healthy in our attitudes toward sex. Books such as *The Joy of Sex* and *More Joy* attest to this. Now that understanding has been broadened, however, it is possible, indeed necessary, to go beyond joy; to go beyond the physical and emotional aspects of sexual union to the ecstasy of union with Divine Power that is centered in every body and throughout the universe.

In Dr. Mumford's view, "The sexual dynamic represents the most significant physical experience that we have at our disposal, and it lies within our power to turn this function into a spiritually regenerative act and a psychologically integrative practice."

The value of his approach is that he makes the spiritual potential of the sexual dynamic accessible to more than the mystic, yogi and occultist. One need not go up to the mountaintop to commune with Divinity: Its temple is the body, Its sacrament the communion between lovers, and that communion involves all the awesome powers of the universe in the microcosm of the lovers.

The once hidden, and forbidden, secret practices of magick are now explicitly revealed. This book traces the ancient practices of Hindu Tantra through the Egyptian, Greek and Hebrew forms where the sexual act is viewed as symbolic of the highest union, oneness with God, to the highest expression of Western sex magick in the Mass of the Holy Ghost.

A psychotherapist trained in Yoga, Dr. Mumford (whose initiated name is Swami Anandakapila) guides the reader through mental and physical exercises aimed at developing psycho-sexual power; he details the various sexual practices and positions that facilitate "psychic short-circuiting" and the arousal of Kundalini, the "Goddess of Life," within the body; and in a chapter subtitled "The Semantics of the Inner Life," he shows how language may be used to break down comfortable categories of reality, inducing a creative autism that unlocks esoteric knowledge and frees the mind to experience enlightenment.

A great advantage of his approach is that he brings the perspective of the East to bear on the newly quickened interest in Western occultism. He shows, for example, the fundamental unity of Tantra with Western Wicca as a magickal religion and way of life-affirmation. And he plumbs the depths of Western sex magick, showing how its techniques culminate in spiritual illumination. While in the Western tradition, sex magick may be employed without an emotional commitment between the partners, in the Tantric use of sex, which is grounded on mutual worship and aimed at altering consciousness, the fire of love is utilized to carry the participants through sexual union to union with the Gods.

Previously published under the title, *Sexual Occultism,* this new edition has been revised and expanded with new materials, including:

- Original photographs of erotic sculptures from Khajuraho in central India to illustrate the Indian concepts of erotic beauty.
- Color photographs of couples engaged in the *Asanas of Love* to illustrate those sexual positions for the arousal of Kundalini in Tantric practice.
- *The Rite of Naked Fire* for use by individuals, couples or groups as a consciousness altering preliminary to individual work or Tantric practice by couples.

Ecstasy Through Tantra is a rare work of beauty, high spirituality, and total practicality—restoring Magick to its sacred place on the altar of sexual union.

Other books by Jonn Mumford

Psychomatic Yoga, Thorsons, 1962
Sexual Occultism, First Edition, Llewellyn Publications, 1975
Sexual Occultism, Second, Revised Edition, Compendium Pty. Ltd., Australia, 1977
Tantrische Sexualmagie, German Edition, Sphinx Verlag, Basel, Switzerland, 1984

About the Author

John Mumford (Swami Anandakapila) has devoted his life to the vast, intricate subject of Tantric Yoga. A disciple of Parahamsa Swami Satyananda Saraswati, Monghyr, Bihar, India, Dr. Mumford originally trained as a psychologist and later as a chiropractor. He now lectures and teaches in Sydney, Australia.

In 1967 he established Australia's first Yoga Teacher's Association, "The Scientific Samkhyan Yoga Association" and commenced training Yoga teachers in anatomy, physiology, psychology and Sanskrit. He conducts classes and seminars across Australia.

In 1961 he wrote *Psychosomatic Yoga* while completing a two-year study period in India. This book has become a standard reference text on Yoga as a method of psycho-physiology.

John Mumford's mastery of Yoga as a psycho-physiological technology has been publicly demonstrated through such controls as cardiac cessation, obliteration of temporal and radial pulses, photographic memory techniques using concentration methods peculiar to Yoga, Khumbhaka or breath retentions in the first five-minute range, Pratyahra (sensory withdrawal), raising pain tolerance and digestive peristalsis control utilizing ground glass as the media. He consistently emphasizes that "Practice without theory is blind and theory without practice is sterile!"

To Write to the Author

If you wish to contact the author or would like more information about this book, please write to the author in care of Llewellyn Worldwide, and we will forward you request. Both the author and publisher appreciate hearing from you and learning of your enjoyment of this book and how it has helped you. Llewellyn Worldwide cannot guarantee that every letter written to the author can be answered, but all will be forwarded. Please write to:

John Mumford
c/o Llewellyn Worldwide
P.O. Box 64383-494, St. Paul, MN 55164-0383, U.S.A.

Please enclose a self-addressed, stamped envelope for reply, or $1.00 to cover costs.
If outside the U.S.A., enclose international postal reply coupon.

Free Catalog from Llewellyn

For more than 90 years Llewellyn has brought its readers knowledge in the fields of metaphysics and human potential. Learn about the newest books in spiritual guidance, natural healing, astrology, occult philosophy and more. Enjoy book reviews, new age articles, a calendar of events, plus current advertised products and services. To get your free copy of *Llewellyn's New Worlds of Mind and Spirit*, send your name and address to:

Llewellyn's New Worlds of Mind and Spirit
P.O. Box 64383-494, St. Paul, MN 55164-0383, U.S.A.

Llewellyn's Tantra & Sexual Arts Series

ECSTASY THROUGH TANTRA

By

Jonn Mumford
(Swami Anandakapila)

1993
Llewellyn Publications
St. Paul, Minnesota 55164-0383, U.S.A.

THIRD REVISED EDITION, 1988
Fourth Printing, 1993

Color photography by Andrew Clarke
Paintings by Martin Cannon
Book design by Terry Buske
Photographs from Khajuraho by Melissa Jade, 1985
Cover design and title by Melissa Jade
Furnishings in color photo sequence from
    L. & A. Copeland and Folk Art
    Warrandyte, Victoria Australia

Library of Congress Cataloging-in-Publication Data
Mumford, John.
    Ecstasy through tantra.

    (Llewellyn's tantra & sexual arts series)
    Bibliography: p.
    1. Sex—Miscellanea. 2. Magic. 3. Tantrism.
I. Title. II. Series.
BF1623.S4M84   1988   133   87-45734
ISBN 0-87542-494-5

Llewellyn Publications
A Division of Llewellyn Worldwide, Ltd.
P.O. 64383, St. Paul, MN 55164-0383

Dedicated to

GURUDEV Paramhansa Swami Satyananda Saraswati

Acknowledgements

I am grateful to *Yoga-Mimamsa Journal,* Lonavla, India for permission to include an extract from Volume XIII, Number 4, January 1971; and to the Theosophical Publishing House, Adyar, Madras, for permission to reprint a passage from *The Hatha Yoga Pradipika.*

Chapter 16 of *The Tree of Life* by Israel Regardie is reproduced by permission of Llewellyn Publications, St. Paul, MN.

My gratitude to Gurudev Paramahansa Satyananda Saraswati, Bihar School of Yoga for the quotations from his *Tantra of Kundalini Yoga* and *Tantra-Yoga Panorama.*

This 3rd Edition has been enhanced by inclusion of Melissa Jade's photographs, and words cannot express my appreciation for her help and patience.

I would also like to express my gratitude to Martin Cannon for his beautiful paintings and to Terry Buske for her design of this book. Thank you to everyone at Llewellyn who helped make this new edition possible.

Contents

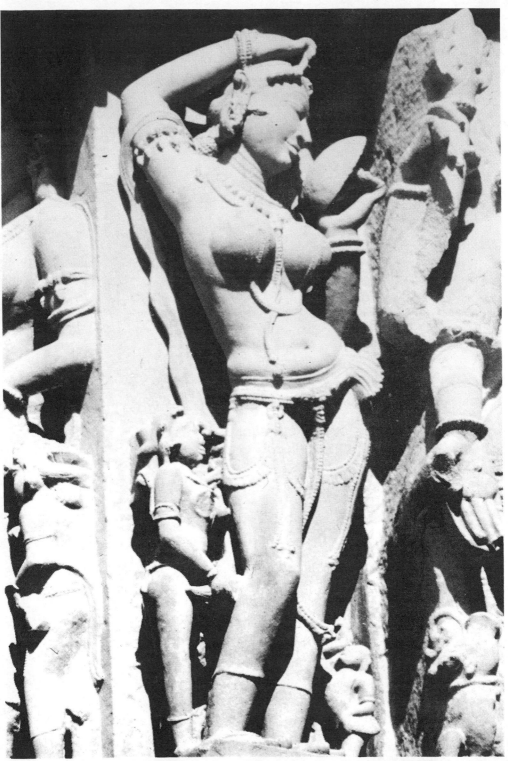

Lady applying vermilion using concave mirror. Lakshmana Temple, Khajuraho, India.

—Introduction—
by
Carl Llewellyn Weschcke

TANTRA—A WORD that is becoming more familiar
to Westerners, but one yet largely misunderstood.
Most of us were first exposed to the word through a
rather popular book published in 1964, *Tantra: The
Yoga of Sex,* by Omar Garrison (Julian Press, New
York). The book was rather a light survey, but it did
introduce the concept of *sex as a religious rite* to a
generation on the verge of the great sexual liberation
that characterized the late 1960's and early 1970's. It
was a book for the times.

   Garrison did give the readers some good tidbits
upon which an edifice of personal experience could
be built, but Tantra is not Yoga, and Tantra is not
limited to "sex" *per se.*

   Many of us believe that Tantra is the oldest single
source of knowledge concerning the energies of the
Mind/Body/Spirit/Soul complex—how old no one
knows—and that it was upon *this* Tantra that the
edifices of Indian Yoga and Chinese Alchemy were
erected.

Yoga and Alchemy—not the pseudo-alchemy of medieval *pre*-science, but the technology for the transformation of the Human into the Divine—are both remarkable and comprehensive methods for the perfection of body and psyche, and the transformation of consciousness. Their extensions lead progressively to the Martial Arts of China and Japan,* to the development of the *Yi King* as a personal tool of knowledge, and to the grand philosophies of the Buddha, Confucius and Lao-tzu.

However, their root source is in Tantra, and Tantra remains their foundation. Today's student of Yoga, or the Martial Arts, or Eastern (or Western) Philosophy, sees only the magnificent edifice, while the foundation is "occult" (i.e. hidden away). It is rather like visiting a beautiful cathedral of wondrous beauty: you can worship therein, you can admire the architecture and glory in the dedication of the craftspeople who built it, and you can study the present-day doctrines of the religion, but you cannot experience their source except by going to the foundations by which the founders themselves entered into living relationship with the Divine.

The edifice itself was built to reflect the needs and culture of a particular moment in history. It may no longer meet the needs of people today, and even though its technology may still be effective, its language may be as archaic as the swords and daggers of martial arts. In the end, Yoga, Tai Chi, Zen, etc. are effective and efficient as physical and mental conditioning programs— *yet their spiritual efficacy requires a lifestyle suited to a culture and time beyond the reach of most people today.*

As Paramahansa Satyananda Saraswati, head of the Bihar (India) School of Yoga, writes (*Tantra-Yoga Panorama,* International Yoga Fellowship Movement, Rajanandgaon, India):

". . . Tantra is meant for the common man and

---

* Dr. Mumford was the first Westerner to correlate the Indian Chakra with the vital striking points of Martial Arts in *Psychosomatic Yoga,* 1962.

Yoga, which is part of Tantra, is meant for an uncommon man. Tantra does not accept any kind of religious, cultural or tribal or national inhibitions.

... this difference which I make between myself and yourself because of the way of life that you lead and the way of life I lead is something which is not in Tantra. I do not want you to make a departure from your status of life, nor do I have any disrespect for your status of life. I think if there is any science, if there is any religion in the world which has respect for human weaknesses, then it is Tantra. Otherwise all religions and all systems of Yoga are intolerant, they cannot understand the laws . . . of natural evolution to which you are subjected, to which I am subjected, to which everybody is subjected and nobody is free from them. . . . Therefore it is said in Tantra, to whichever religion you may belong, or to whichever ethical beliefs you may belong, or whatever may be your way of eating and living, you don't make a departure from your status in life . . . Tantra accepts that three billion people cannot belong to only one range of life."

What then, is Tantra? Tantra is a spiritual *Science* involving "methods of going into the subconscious mind and diving deep into the unconscious mind . . . to clear up your personality, your deep-rooted complexes, going to correct your behavior, is going to rehabilitate you psychologically, and physically." Tantra is also Kundalini Yoga, and "The purpose of Kundalini Yoga is to awaken the powerful consciousness or the psychic consciousness in man in order to make it possible for him to have the vision of a greater reality in himself."*

---

* *Ibid.*

Tantra is the science, and includes many techniques dealing with Mantra, Yantra, Mandala, Yoganidra, Asana, Pranayama, etc. In other words, it includes the use of special sounds and words, diagrams and visualizations, sacred pictures, guided meditation and self-hypnosis, postures and movement, breath control, and all the techniques used in all religious, magical and growth disciplines. It is the use of such techniques that can lead to living experience with Divinity.

As a science, Tantra is universal. The various techniques that we find today in Yoga, or in mental and spiritual systems of discipline and religious practice, are all edifices built upon that fundamental root-knowledge whose origins are timeless. Tantra is also the name we give to the "Old Religion" of the East, and many of us believe it is essentially identical with aspects of both Wicca and Kabbalah in the West—but with Tantra we have a relative continuity of knowledge down to the present day, unlike that in the West—largely lost through persecutions, first by the Church, and then by 19th century "Scientism."

Much of this Eastern Tantra has become obscure if not lost, and its revival and recovery is as much part of the New Age (that began perhaps in January 1962,* when the Earth entered Aquarius) as is the conviction that peace is both possible and vital, that every life can have personal meaning, and that life is everywhere and in all things. Since then we have seen a total rebirth of Tantric Science—with new study, research, and practice of all aspects of Yoga, Mysticism, Meditation, the Martial Arts, Magick, Metaphysics, Wicca and Shamanism. All of these are but techniques to accomplish one thing:

> *The essential message of Tantra is "Look within—find, and express Divinity." Learn to invoke God and Goddess within yourselves, learn to use the creative power of the Divinity within to transform Body and Soul, and to improve daily life.*

---

* *Ibid.*

Tantra provides a foundation for contemporary men and women to understand their role in a New Age. It shows the way by which we may gain the necessary vision to solve both personal and planet-wide problems. It gives us the means to penetrate to the core essentials, and make contemporary adaptations of all the yogas and religions and psychologies that are our human heritage. It opens the way to finding "Light Within" and applying "Power Without."

Yes, Tantra is the science of consciousness—but its first principles are easily applied because it recognizes and accepts the structure of the human psyche and builds upon the most powerful experience available to the common man and woman: LOVE. Yes, sex too, but not as "the yoga of sex" which suggests more in the way of sexual athletics than the powerful dynamo of life-force that not only unites Man and Woman and reproduces the race, but that awakens—even if but for a moment—the "sleeping giant" which is the nine-tenths of human potential that lies dormant in most of us.

Crowley said "Love is the Law, Love under Will." Love is the answer to contemporary ills, and it is the energies aroused through magical love, *guided by Will,* that provide solutions to problems.

Love, Law, Will. Three words with special meaning. But there's nothing complicated in these words. We *live* them all the time. There's no escaping the "Law" as it is intended here, for it is *the Laws of Nature* that is meant— and Love is the key to recognizing those laws and living by them. "Will" is not a real problem, for all it means, really, is to be aware and to act with purpose and meaning *in the expression of Love and recognition of Law.*

What Tantra gives us is the key to bringing into the sexual relationship that which is promised in nearly every religious rite sanctifying marriage: *holiness.*

Tantra knows that Sexual Energy is Feminine—it is the Goddess, the Mother, Holy Earth. All Life as we know it is of Her. When we do not live "within Her," we abuse the

Goddess. Love *is* the Law, for with love we cannot abuse the Mother. Every person, male and female both, is a "channel" between God and Goddess—between Sky and Earth—and as we awaken to the Divinity within and open the channels for the ebb and flow of Divine Energies, we accelerate the evolution of consciousness, the healing of the Earth and all within Her (including Humanity), and open the way for the New Age.

What is easier than finding God in the man you love, or the Goddess in the woman you love? Express the Divinity that is within you, and adore the Divinity within your beloved! Allow yourself, at the very deepest levels of the psyche, to respond to your beloved's *invocation of the Divine* within you! Give pleasure to your beloved, and learn how to give greater pleasure! Study loving, practice love, be loved!

Study Sex! To use contemporary terminology: Plug In, Power Up, Switch On, and Open the Channels! Sex is part of Love, just as Yoga is part of Tantra. Sex is part of all we do, for polarity is the condition of existence, and sex connects the poles—*Sex restores Wholeness, Love gives it Holiness.*

The concept of Tantra might be paraphrased thus:

> We are created as "Gods in potentials," or—if your prefer—"in the image of our Creator." "Male and Female created He Them." Tantra says that we have, in our brain and psycho-spiritual apparatus, a vast treasure trove of undeveloped abilities. In the normal course of human evolution, we will grow, develop, and utilize this potential—in millions of years! Tantra offers a system to speed up that transformation in the entire structure of the brain, to attain full illumination and manifestation as soon as possible.

TAN-TRA means to *expand* and to *liberate*. It is through the fulfillment of our potential that we become free. Growth is the obligation placed upon us by Life itself—for no other purpose can we perceive in all creation. Growth is the key to a happy, healthful and successful life. The ability to continue growing is the key to extended life.

The ultimate goal is to *Connect Up*. In Hinduism, Shiva is the name of God, and Shakti is His consort. But Shiva also means "Supreme Awareness" which is said to reside at the Crown Chakra, while Shakti is the "Divine Power" residing at the perineum. "Yoga" (any technology based on Tantra) means to join the two, to unite Unconscious with Super-conscious. Sex awakens the Divine Power, and magical loving unites Shakti with Shiva.

Another way to explore Tantra is to realize that *pleasure is experienced in the brain*—and orgasm can be directed to the brain if the foreplay is extended long enough! Are we saying anything different in this paragraph than we did in the previous one? No, it's just another way of expressing the technology.

Does it matter so much how we describe a process as it does that we proceed with it: *to Love One Another!*

This book is about "magical loving"—making sex into a religious rite, into a technique of growth in consciousness, into the glue that makes the parts whole.

People who practice magical loving say that "every sexual union produces a Magical Child." That's to say that every union of Man and Woman is magical, and produces something composed of these parts. Express the Divinity within in your Loving Union, and you will manifest Divinity in your lives and in all that you do.

No sweeter message, nor any more simple: "Love One Another"!

—Carl Llewellyn Weschcke
Publisher

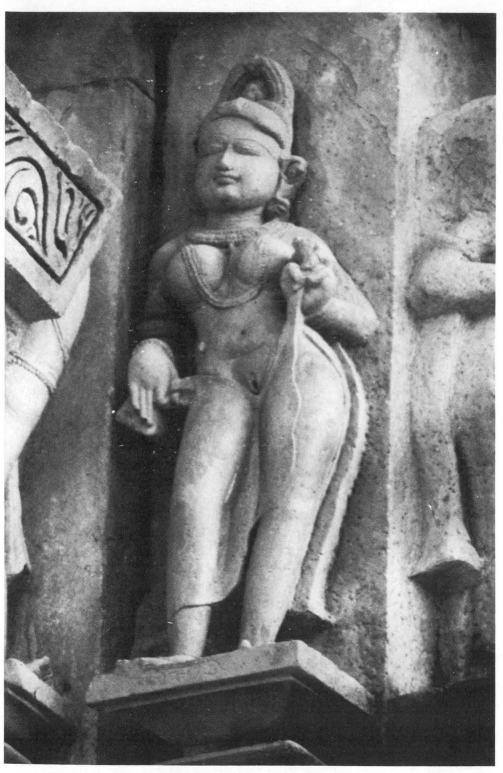

Lakshmana Temple, Khajuraho.

Preface

I HAVE COMPILED the material for *Ecstasy Through Tantra* over many years involving various phases in the evolution of my personal research and growth. The "sexual" implications inherent in mysticism are emphasized for the enjoyment of those who are occult epicureans or gourmets of the esoteric. It is my profound hope that encouragement will be given to all, through this book, for utilizing the sexual dimension as a key unlocking joyous power.

Far greater minds than mine have acknowledged the truism that the relationship between mankind and the Absolute is either an analogue to, or a projection of, the sexual-emotional activity of human beings. The testament of this is found in a common motif, appearing in sources as diverse as the *Songs of Solomon* and twentieth-century Freudian Psychoanalysis.

Readers wishing confirmation of the historical reality of Tantra and scholastic evidence for the material presented herein, are referred to Zimmer's *Philosophies of India,* Eliade's *Yoga: Immortality and Freedom* and Swami Agehananda Bharati's *The Tantric Tradition.* I have deliberately avoided giving copious footnotes and references, preferring to concern myself with the "spirit" rather than the "letter" of the law.

Those desiring further information concerning the practice of Western magic as an integrating system are advised to obtain Louis T. Culling's masterpiece, *The Complete Magick Curriculum of the Secret Order of G∴B∴G∴*, which I consider the best practical working manual ever published.

To be completely satisfied with a purely scientific appraisal of what has variously been termed "the Great Work," "the White Blaze of Kether," "Samadhi," and "Nirvana" is a demonstration of rustic puerility by comparison with the creative value of the actual subjective experience.

In the final analysis I maintain that occultism (i.e., the study of the hidden or obscure) is the greatest adventure on which humans are capable of embarking. In the history of *Homo sapiens,* artistic and religious expression have been the product of Hermetic inner moments, and this shall always be so until the day our planet falls back into the womb of the Sun furnace that gave us birth.

—Jonn Mumford

Sex Magic

THE WESTERN MAGICAL tradition has a definite teaching concerning "sex magic." This doctrine, although similar to Tantra, sometimes differs in the goal sought. Power, not spiritual consciousness, is often the object of the magician who practices libidinous ritual. This is so frequently the case that Dion Fortune unequivocally stated that sexual acts used as an adjunct to ceremonial magic are tantamount to black magic and the practitioner automatically defines himself as a follower of the left-hand path. *Few modern occultists would agree with her simplistic viewpoint, for it is the end sought, not the means used, which determines the shade of magic.*

By defining magic we can understand fully the implications of sex magic. "Magic" is a word of Persian origin, the root being *magi,* meaning a Persian priest, an enchanter, a wise man who interprets dreams, a fire worshiper. Related concepts are *magister,* a teacher or master, and *magus,* a magician of adept standard. Reference to any good dictionary reveals a

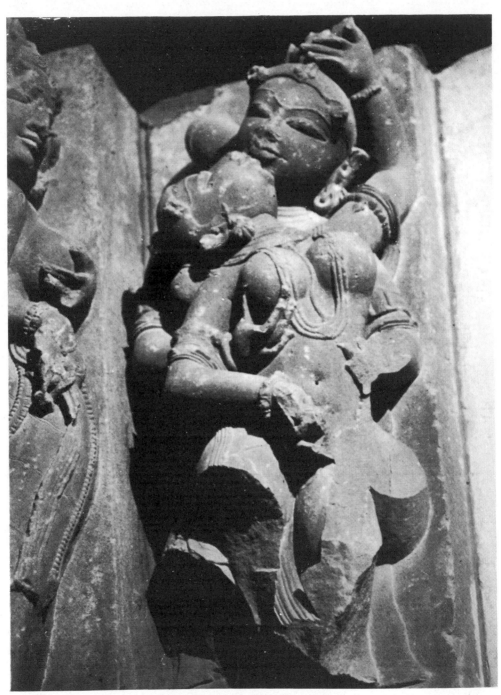

Chitragupta Temple, Khajuraho.

scattering of words using the Greek prefix *mag* meaning "great," similar to the Sanskrit *maha*, as in *maharaja* (great king). Such words with magical connotations include *magistrate* (a ruler), *magnate* (a great man), *magnificent* (doing great things), *magniloquence* (elevated language; facility with mantra, words of power), *magnanimity* (greatness of mind), and finally *magnetism*. (Consider how often Mesmerism, odic fluid, orgone, prana, aura and polarity are basic concepts prevalent in magical doctrines of psychic magnetism.)

Aleister Crowley stated that magic is the science of causing changes to occur in conformity with the will. Although we tend not to view it as such, *everything we do is "magic," for whenever we will something and cause it to materialize, a magical act has been performed;* i.e., a change occurs in conformity with the will. Because most aspects of our life appear to have distinct cause-and-effect relationships, we take them for granted. If the causal threads are tenuous or even invisible, we may suddenly take notice. When a hitherto healthy African or Aborigine boy dies for no other reason than because the witch doctor "pointed" the bone, then the thin veneer of educated reason may be pushed aside by sudden feelings from primitive layers of our being concerned with witchcraft and the supernatural. This, in turn, may be counteracted by rationalizations such as "it is psychosomatic," and if we successfully calm ourselves down, we once again can sink back into the rut of everyday thinking and feeling.

Sex magic rests upon the fact that the most important psychophysiological event in the life of a human being is an orgasm. *Sex magic is the art and science of utilizing sexual experience for the concrete materialization of desire and the expansion of the inner life.*

Successful sex magic involves an interplay of four factors:

- All aspects of extrasensory perception are heightened during sexual excitation. The non-verbal communication and responsiveness of partners attuned to each others' needs during love-making is one example.

- Immediately before, during and after the climax, the mind is in a state of hypersensitivity, soaking up all suggestions like a sponge. Many sexual problems, frigidity and impotence in particular, have their origin in a careless comment uttered by a partner prior to or just after the climax. A person engaged in intercourse is highly vulnerable to positive or negative influences.

- Consistency of peak sexual sensations facilitates access to the unconscious realms, or the "astral" worlds of the occultist and the *Kundalini* arousal of the Tantrist. Prevalence of postcoital dreams, visions and kaleidoscopic effects provides ample evidence that this is so.

- During orgasm many people have experienced, at least once, a true Samadhi involving timelessness and a total dissolution of the ego, accompanied by subjective sensations of being absorbed by their partner.

Just as many aspects of Hindu occultism have had their inception in Tantra, so much of Western occultism has derived from the Semitic triad (Judaism, Christianity, and Islam). The Semitic triad, in turn, has been influenced by the even older Egyptian culture.

Probably the best illustration that hidden aspects of sex were recognized in the ancient world can be seen in the Nile Valley civilization and its adaptation of the Ankh or Crux Ansata as a religious emblem. This Tau cross, surmounted by an oval, symbolized eternal life and resurrection. The

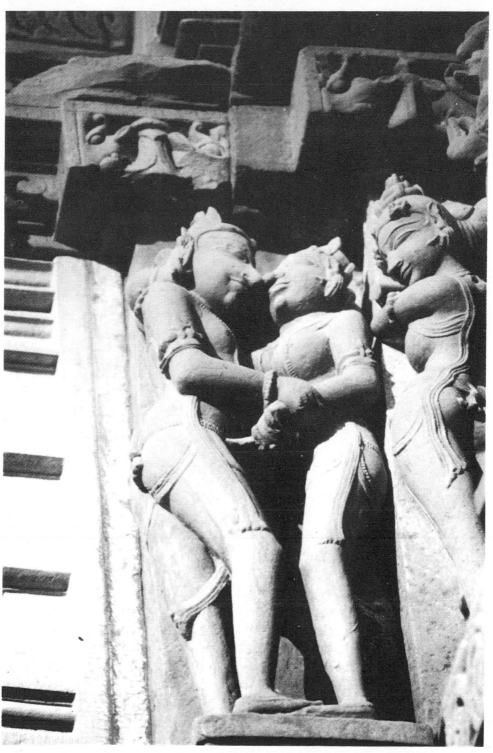

Nose Touching, Chitragupta Temple, Khajuraho.

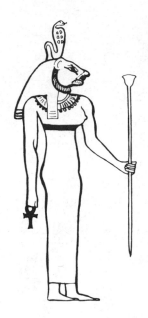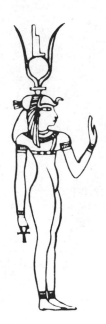

Ankh is found in the hands of the Gods, upon tomb walls and sarcophagi lids and placed in the withered, wrapped hands of the deceased. This glyph was placed wherever desire for immortality was implied.

The Egyptian myth of the resurrection of Osiris by his son Horus, and the impregnation of Isis through magic rites performed upon her husband's corpse to reanimate the penis, are legends summing up the secret nature of the Ankh. Although Egyptologists favor the opinion that the Ankh was originally a graphic picture of a man or a sandal thong, certain Western fraternities have always taught that it is a vivid representation of the male phallus (vertical line) united with the female genitalia (vagina and uterus, as represented by the horizontal line and oval). *Thus, the Ankh was the symbol of eternity as perpetuated through the sexual activity of mankind.*

It is suggested that the priests of Isis originally drew the Ankh in two parts, with the vertical line separated from the horizontal line and oval. Later it became necessary to conceal

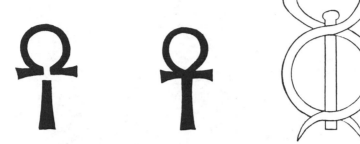

the esoteric meaning of the Ankh and they converted it to an exoteric symbol by representing the two sections as joined, in the form now known to Western archaeologists.

It is probable that the Egyptians exerted a strong influence over Jewish occultism, and therefore we may conjecture a certain pattern in the development of Western mysticism as having its original roots along the banks of the Nile. The Egyptian priests may have passed directly to the Hebrews the tradition of hidden teachings associated with the *Shekinah*. "Shekinah" is a Hebrew word meaning "the Dwelling," the visible presence of the divine. This refers to the descent and manifestation of God among men. This sacred presence occurs only under conditions of special holiness, and, like *Shakti,* is considered in some Kabbalistic teachings as a revealing of divinity personified by the eternal feminine.

A. E. Waite, writing in his book *The Holy Kabbalah,* suggests that Jewish esotericism considers the conjugal relationship to be a most suitable time for the descent of the Shekinah upon the man and woman. As in Tantra, the act of intercourse is symbolical of a higher unity (oneness of God) ritually manifested on the material plane by physical union. *This results in a transmutation of the couple through the automatic invocation of the Shekinah,*

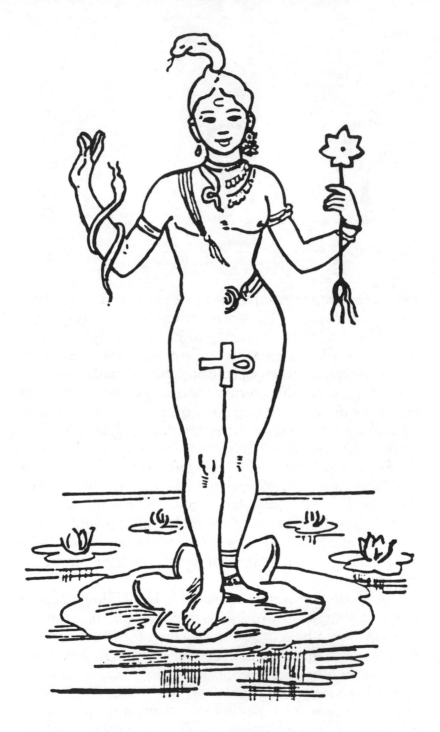

Ardanari-Iswara

which falls upon them like a sacred mantle or cloak. Some schools of thought look upon this Kabbalistic doctrine as the father of the comparatively exoteric Catholic ritual of the mass with its magical act of Transubstantiation.

Again, as in Tantra, the physical bodies of the participants are regarded as *altars* or tabernacles (the word means a "tent," implying an enveloping auric field) made ready by the pure intent of the couple and sanctified by the presence of the Shekinah at the moment of orgasm. Mr. Waite gives a Latin quotation which is a most explicit statement that the Holy Spirit (Shekinah) exists within the genital parts. This is reminiscent of a popular Buddhist Tantra quotation that enlightenment resides in the sexual parts of women ("Buddhatvam Yosityonisamasritam").

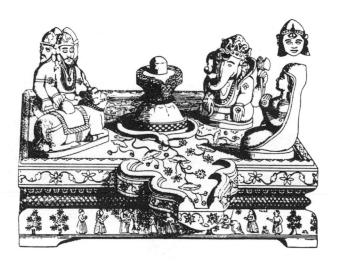

In addition to the contributions of the Egyptians and Jews to the Western tradition of sex magic, we must mention another source. The Greeks believed that originally man was a hermaphrodite—or bisexual, androgynous being—created by the God Zeus as a plaything. One day, Zeus, the king of the Gods, became angry with the miserable creation on Earth and threw down a thunderbolt which split the animal into two halves, the prototypes of male and female. Since this event, man has been plagued with a feeling of incompleteness and unbearable loneliness as he searches the Earth for his other half. It is only in cohabitation or sexual yoking that he finds "wholeness." ("Holiness" is linguistically closely allied, and in Middle English "whole" was spelled "hole" with "holy" as the derivative.)

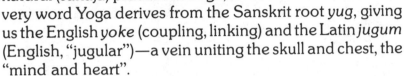

Intercourse is the first and most natural (sahaja) practice in Yoga, for the very word Yoga derives from the Sanskrit root *yug*, giving us the English *yoke* (coupling, linking) and the Latin *jugum* (English, "jugular")—a vein uniting the skull and chest, the "mind and heart".

Perhaps the most important synthesis of Western Tantric concepts came through the formation of the O.T.O., or "Ordo Templi Orientis," around the turn of the last century. The O.T.O. was a Western occult fraternity which based its teachings upon the occult sexology of both East and West. Only initiated members knew that the secret meaning of the initials O.T.O. was "Order to Ov." *To ov* is a Greek term meaning an emanation of liquid or astral fire. At the physical level this was a direct reference to semen, and at the psychic level indicated kundalini, which is the alchemical titration of seminal or vaginal secretions, according to Tantric teaching.

The practical work of the O.T.O. combined Western ceremonial magic with Tantric sexology. Thus, a IX° ritual or act was synonymous with sex magic. The magician who performed such a ritual attempted to produce a magical result by the ceremonial performance of a heterosexual act. Other degrees dealt with autosexual and homosexual magic, as it was recognized that any sexual activity, whether normal or so-called deviate, released copious quantities of psychic energy into the body and surrounding environment.

All that was required was the tapping and controlling of this force for magical purposes, rather than the permitting of its dissipation in the usual manner.

This type of thaumaturgy might involve the consecration of a special temple by the use of the pentagram ritual* and other techniques of Occidental magic, or it might simply involve an act of concentration by the practitioner at the moment of climax, with the object of influencing another person telepathically.

A very special example of this is known as "The Mass of the Holy Ghost." This is a Mass in which the elements of Transubstantiation are the fluids secreted from the bodies of the couple participating. Western sexual alchemy, like Tantra, is literal "feeding on love." This ceremony is not a parody of the Catholic Mass and is similar only in aim; i.e., Transubstantiation. The Mass may be performed with the intention of creating an occult elixir of life, for the magnetizing of a special talisman, or simply as a method of incarnating one of the Godheads from the Egyptian or Greek pantheon.

The best description of this Mass, which I do not consider to be an act of the left-hand path, is found in Israel Regardie's *The Tree of Life,* Chapter Sixteen (see Appendix A). He explains the details, couched in alchemical terms, for those who can read between the lines.

Western Tantra, similar to some Eastern aspects (Prayoga and Strickmarni), is greatly concerned with the use of body substances for occult and alchemical purposes. One branch of this frankly venereal magic composes potent aphrodisiacs, perfumes and draughts, utilizing sympathetic magic and the Laws of Correspondence as revealed by the Tree of Life.

The key secret of the Western tradition lies in the demonstration that the sexual function has deeper implications than procreation. Twentieth-century life builds up

---

*See any text on Western ritual magic, such as Regardie's *The Golden Dawn* or Kraig's *Modern Magick.*

psychic tension, and the correct, occult use of sex may act as a safety valve for such accumulated nervous energy. Individuals who become fully aware of each other's needs in this regard may develop an extremely practical outlook upon the whole concept of sexual relationships.

The sexual dynamic represents the most significant physical experience the occultist has at his disposal, and it lies within his power to turn this function into a spiritually regenerative act and a psychologically integrative practice.

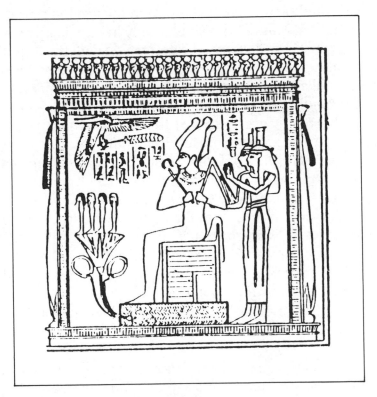

Osiris

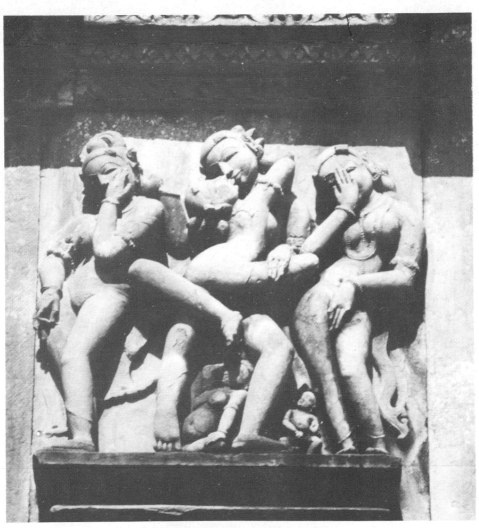

Vishvanath Temple, Khajuraho.

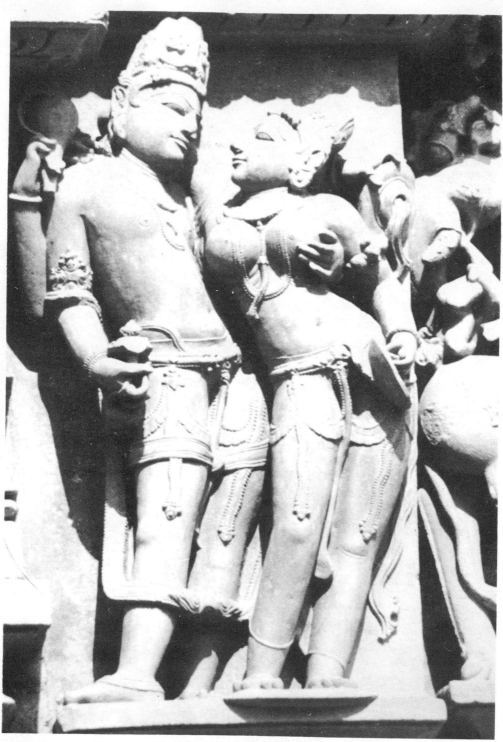

Vishnu and Lakshmi, Parsvanath Temple, Khajuraho.

Tantra

INDIA IS A land of physical contrasts and philosophical paradoxes. The soil, soaked in the sweat of a culture far older than our civilization, nurtures practices as divergent as the covert rituals of the Tantric adepts and the overt worship of the Shiva Linga. Hindu and Occidental alike conceive magic smouldering in the magician's phallic "wand." As D. H. Lawrence suggested, man is possessed of a rod connecting him to the stars (Chakras). Indian philosophy has encompassed every aspect of existence, including the relationship of the sexual impulse to the harnessing of occult forces and attainment of self-realization.

Among Indian philosophers there is a major conflict in their attitude toward sex in general and women in particular. "See every woman as filled with urine and feces" is the advice of a purportedly saintly personality in northern India. "Women are the Gods, women are life, women are adornment. Be ever among women in thought" are the words attributed to the Buddha in the Cina-Cara-Sara Tantric text.

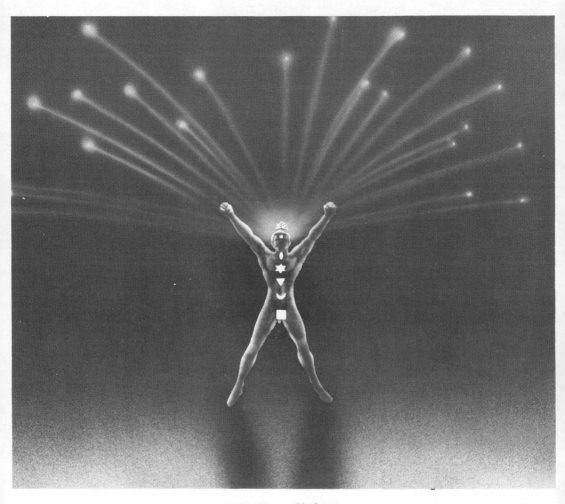

The Seven Chakras

The divergence indicated in these two quotations involves not only the question of sexual feeling as potential occult energy, but also the problem of the best attitude toward women as a vivid symbol of the primal power of sexual manifestation.

The Indian rishi has always associated sexual activity with the female, particularly the aspect personified in the worship of Shiva's spouse in her varied guises as the blood-thirsty Kali, the warlike Durga, the lovely Uma and gentle Parvati.

How did this attribution of everything sexual to the feminine arise? It was inherent in the roots of Aryan-Dravidian society and perhaps was an indirect acknowledgment of the now gnomic expression in Western sociology: "The female of the species is biologically and psychologically superior."

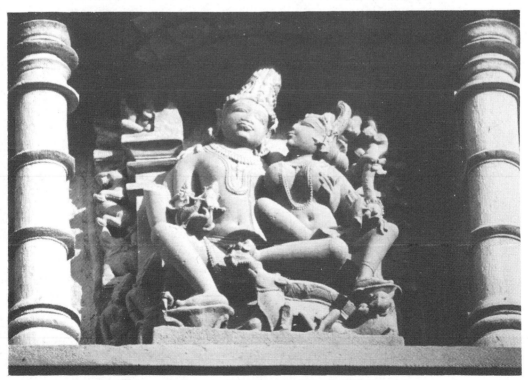

Shiva and Parvati, Chitragupta Temple, Khajuraho.

Five thousand years ago the original inhabitants of the Indus Valley were a dark-skinned people now known as Dravidians. P. Thomas in his *Kama Kalpa* states that there is evidence indicating that early Indian society was originally matriarchal, later becoming patriarchal under Vedic influence. This may well be so, for the indigenous religion of the Dravidians before the Aryan invasions c. 1,000 B.C. was Tantra.

Tantra (literally "loom, thread, web, ritual, doctrine") is considered most suitable for this Dark Age, the Kali Yuga, because it directly recognizes woman as the highest materialization of the Godhead. One of the minor Upanishads echoes Tantra, stating, "The vulva is an altar and the pubic hairs the flames upon the altar."

The concepts of Tantra have so influenced Indian culture that despite a Hindu society which is distinctly patriarchal, Westerners are even today prone to differentiate

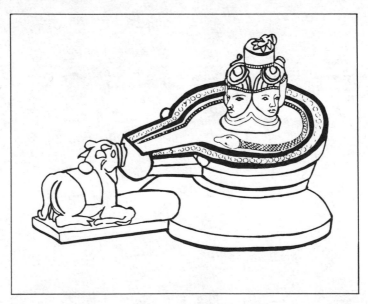

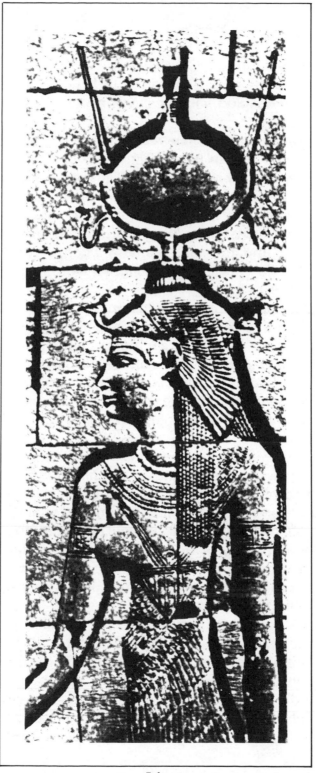

Isis

between Hinduism and Christianity by noting that Christians speak of the fatherhood of God while Hindus speak of the motherhood of God, with the "Divine Mother" as the cosmic archetype.

Personifying as female that which is manifest power and energy is not an idea exclusive to Eastern thought. Buried deep in the racial unconscious of Western man is also the concept of feminine power. We need only recall our contemporary habit of assigning female names to hurricanes, a custom probably inherited from Greek mythology, and the three female witches collectively called "Furies" (hence such English words as "fierce" and "furious").

Indian philosophy contains antagonistic viewpoints regarding the use or nonuse of sexual activity for spiritual gain. The older Dravidian Tantric teaching is concerned with the attainment of freedom (Moksha) through the utilization of sex as a cosmic springboard while later Aryan Yoga schools introduced the concept of sexual celibacy, or Brahmacharya, as an absolute necessity for realization (Samadhi).

Tantra is the positive Indian teaching concerning the physical manifestations of sex. Tantra, although often badly misunderstood, is still the most potent and vital stream of Indian philosophy. Hinduism may be the mother of all religions, but Tantra is the mother of Indian metaphysics. Indeed, a contemporary Yogi, Swami Satyananda of Bihar, maintains that Tantra, not Samkhya, is the philosophical matrix out of which Yoga grew.

Semen, or Bindu, is held to be the true elixir of life by Yoga and Tantric schools alike. The Hatha Yogin looks upon Brahmacharya as essentially a means of conserving his semen and thus preserving his physical body from the vicissitudes of time. Ayurvedic medicine (an empirical system of Hindu surgery and pharmacology still practiced in modern India alongside Western medicine) claims that some forty drops of blood are required to manufacture one drop of semen, and he who would prolong his life must prevent the loss of this iridescent fluid.

For the Hindu, semen equals distilled blood, and to some extent Western biochemistry corroborates this attitude with the discovery that fresh semen contains liberal quantities of calcium, iron, phosphorus and vitamin C, all of which are essential micronutrients in the human body. Semen even possesses antibiotic properties, according to research workers at Hebrew University Medical School, with a particularly effective action upon Staphlyococcus Aureas, or "Golden Staph" (the causative organisms of some minor skin infections such as boils).

The Tantric facial pack par excellence is liberal quantities of fresh, warm semen spread upon the skin, with special attention to the oily areas of the forehead and nose. As the semen dries it closes the pores with an astringent

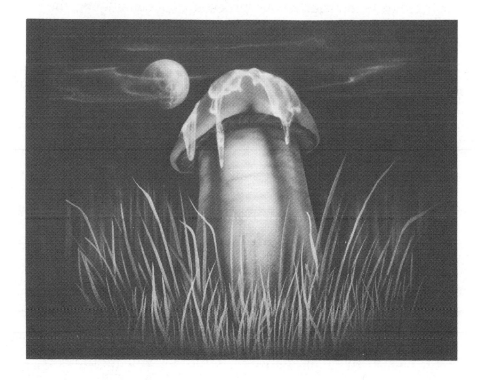

action and tightens the wrinkles, feeds the skin cells and thus leaves the face rejuvenated and smooth.

It is no surprise to the Tantrist when theologian John Allegro (author of *The Sacred Mushroom*) reveals that the word "Christ" is a Greek derivation from an early Sumerian root meaning "smeared with semen." Indeed the neophytes ("new plants") of the Greek mystery schools had their growth accelerated through initiation by anointment with an unguent composed of semen.

The secrets of Tantra are really secretions generated in the cavities (caves) of the bodily temple.

Originally the Hatha Yogin prevented the escape of his seed by celibacy in its strictest interpretation. Tantra, however, has always taught that certain definite advantages accrue from intercourse, the most important being the exchange of positive and negative pranic or subtle energies between the nervous systems of the male and female. This is held to be a regenerative process, especially when the male is able either to prevent the ejaculation of semen at the precise moment of experiencing his own orgasm or, alternatively, to reabsorb his ejaculated essence from the vaginal communion cup of his partner.

It must be emphasized that there is not an iota of medical, physiological, or biochemical evidence *that preventing emission of semen during the male orgasm prolongs life or rejuvenates the body.* This is true in spite of a plethora of contemporary books on Taoism and Yoga suggesting otherwise. Although semen does contain fructose, mineral and vitamin nutrients, the amount is absurdly small in terms of the body reserves. Any intelligent reader, using a calculator and consulting a standard reference (such as *Scientific Tables,* 7th edition, published by Ciba-Geigy Limited, Basle, Switzerland) can quickly establish, as an example, that an average ejaculation of 5 mls. (1 teaspoon) will result in the loss of minimal nutrients.

The concept that men lose energy by ejaculation is a leftover from ancient Indian, Chinese and Mediaeval

European neuroticism. The true value of occasional use of "retrograde ejaculation" methods has to do with inducing an intensified, altered state of consciousness in the male, facilitating magical visualization procedures. The effects are psychic and psychological.

Variations of seminal retention techniques sometimes enhance the possibility of men having multiple orgasms, just as stimulation of trigger points for the Swadhisthana Chakra ('G-spot') may allow some women to experience ejaculation. Neither male multiple orgasms nor female ejaculation constitutes a test of "sexual success"—they merely represent extra-dimensional aspects within a wide spectrum of normal human sexual response.

The first technique, stopping the ejaculation at orgasm, is indigenous to both Tantra and Chinese Taoism. Pressure is exerted on a vital point ("marma") termed Yoni Nadi, which corresponds to the origin of the vessel of conception in Chinese acupuncture. This effectively blocks the tube conveying semen to the penis, much as stepping on a garden hose will stop the flow of water. It is such an effective method of birth control that young people in Mao's China are still taught "Coitus Obstructus," as it is called in Western medicine. The classical Siva Samhita textbook of Hatha Yoga refers to this practice as the frustrating of the mingling of Sun and Moon by "Sahajoli."

We teach the exact Tantric method of adjusting the pressure; it should be remarked that several Hatha Yoga postures (including Siddhasana) in which the heel is pressed hard into the perineum are designed to inhibit seminal flow in a less perfect fashion.

The second method, exclusively Hindu in origin, is the notorius Vajroli (penis) Mudra (gesture). In the Siva Samhita it is called Amaroli. This technique is based upon the startling discovery of Hatha adepts that isolation of the rectus abdominus (a muscle on the anterior abdominal wall, extending from the lower end of the breast bone to the pubic bone) will induce a semi-vacuum in the bowel and bladder. Normally, conscious control of this muscle is difficult, and the Yogin learns to tense it at will by an exercise called Nauli. By creating a partial vacuum in the bladder, the Yogin actually sucks his ejaculated semen back within the urethra (the tube conveying urine and semen through the penis), where it is subsequently reabsorbed by the capillaries in the epithelial lining of the urethra. This effectively returns psychic and chemical elements to the circulation, including tinctures distilled in the alchemical retort of the vagina. Vajroli Mudra is the ultimate in physiological recycling.

The preliminary training for Vajroli Mudra involves tactfully inserting a silver catheter or pipe into the urethra as far as the bladder. With one end of the pipe immersed in a bowl of liquid, the adept performs Madhyama (central control) Nauli and, focusing his attention, literally "wills" the fluid up the catheter, through the penis and into the bladder. Much depends upon the intensity of concentra-

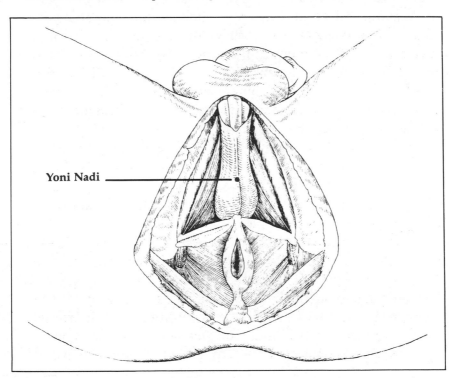

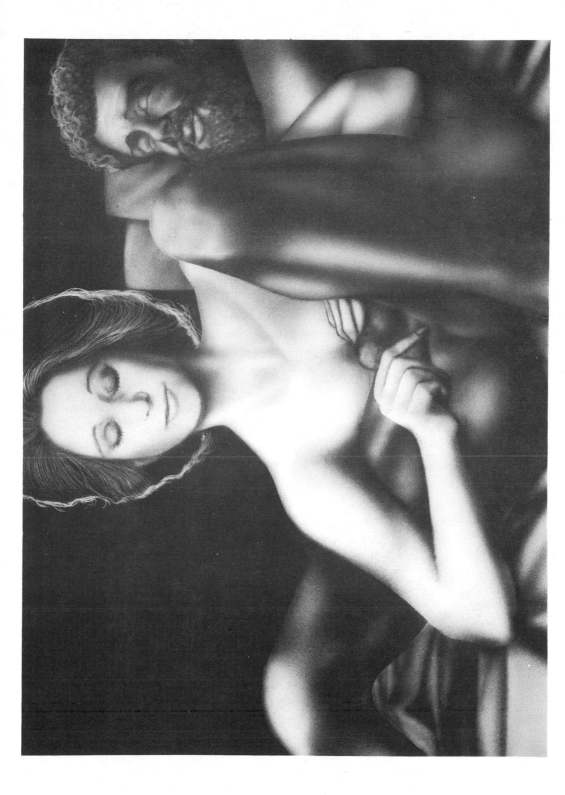

tion, because Vajroli Mudra is an exercise in "mind" over "matter." At an advanced stage the tube is dispensed with.

Greater control is achieved by mastering aspiration of fluids in order of increasing specific gravity, commencing with water and progressing through milk, oil, honey and mercury. It need hardly be emphasized that the risk of internal rupture and cystitis (bladder infection) is high, thus discouraging the average Western student. The correct method of performing Vajroli Mudra is transmitted from mouth to ear by Guru to Chela; when initiated, I was shown a special way of injecting air into the bladder to facilitate the uptake of solutions.

The object of Vajroli Mudra is not merely the recapturing of seminal emissions after climax but the mixing and absorption of a Tantric elixir compounded of male Bindu fortified with hormonally rich vaginal secretions that appear only under conditions of unutterable ecstasy.

Not all masters of Vajroli engage in the practice for psychophysical rejuvenation. As recently as 1971 a bitter comment appeared in the January *Yoga-Mimamsa* (a journal devoted to scientific and philosophico-literary research in Yoga), warning that yogis existed who exploited ignorant villagers by pretending they had purified themselves so thoroughly that even their urine burned as oil. According to Drs. Bhole, M.D., and Karambelker, Ph.D., in "Studies on Sub-atmospheric Pressure Changes in Yoga Practices, III": "Some Yogis exploit the masses through this practice, by claiming that their urine has been purified to such an extent that a cotton wick could be kept burning in it. In fact they suck oil into their bladder beforehand and later pass it as urine in front of the masses. Such and other deceptions go on in the name of Yoga."

Hatha Yoga schools have long been concerned with the possibility of arousing a residue of energy said to be locked within the body. This force is called Kundalini (literally "coiled," implying the power inherent in a compressed spring), and certain techniques will release Kundalini up a central psychic tube termed Shushumna. Shushumna is probably the equivalent of a fluid-filled cavity, the canalis centralis, in the center of the eighteen or so inches of spinal cord.

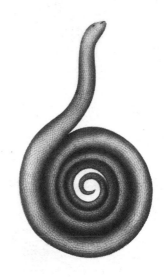

Kundalini wells up in Shushumna when the subsidiary energies in auxiliary psychic nerves, Ida and Pingala (related to the sensory and motor tracts running up and down the spinal cord) cease flowing. Ida, traditionally, is to the left of Shushumna, and Pingala is on the right, reminiscent of the twin chain of sympathetic ganglia in Western anatomy. Some traditions use celibacy as a prerequisite for the building up of sufficient psychic pressure or steam to clear Shushumna and arouse Kundalini. The semen is gradually converted to Ojas, or purified quintessence, which in turn constitutes the basic fuel stoking Kundalini. As Kundalini flows up Shushumna to the brain, various psychic centers, or Chakras, unfold.

Tantra has taken this hypothesis a step further by postulating that all sexual experience automatically arouses Kundalini, and hence a deep spiritual state will ensue from conscious recognition of this process. The woman's body represents the psychic tube Ida, and is a natural channel for negative (apanic) Moon (chandra) energy. The man's body functions as Pingala, a psychic conduit for positive (pranic) Sun (surya) power. At the moment of orgasm, two bodies fuse momentarily on a psychic plane, and the energy of this fusion is focused in the middle channel, Shushumna. The ascent of Kundalini commences, accompanied by the mutual opening of the Chakras, or autonomic nerve plexuses,

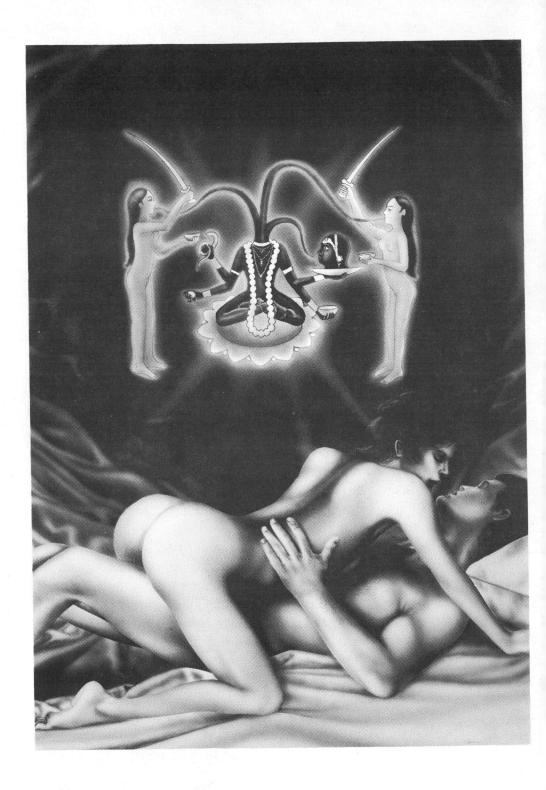

in each participant. One subjective result and test of successful Tantric intercourse is an aftermath of psychedelic visions and color swirls, indicative of the overflow of the unconscious (Kundalini) onto conscious planes.

Tantra was the first school which taught the later Vedantic secret that "Man is God." A couple approaching each other in the sexual embrace tacitly recognize this

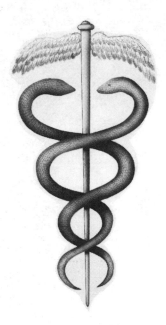

philosophical truth. The woman sees her lover as Krishna and the man sees in her the incarnation of Radha. A God and Goddess unite and transcendental bliss is achieved, using the physical mechanism as a lever.

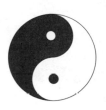

This particular attitude of Tantra has exerted its influence on Buddhism. The Mahayana doctrine of Mahasujha (great delight) is a Buddhist teaching which supports the validity of sexual union as a means of realization. Yab-Yum (Tibetan) and Yang-Ying (Chinese) symbolize this mystery of existence manifested through

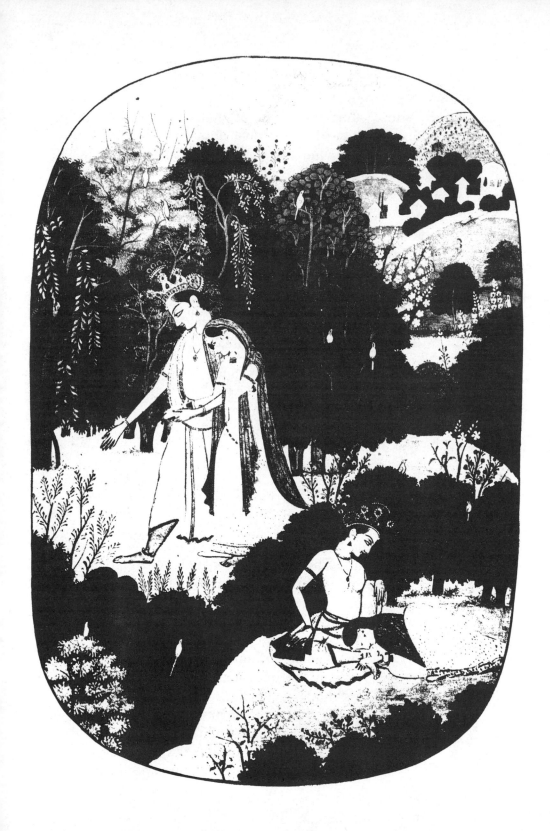

the union of two mind-body complexes producing bliss (Ananda) in the act of intercourse (Maithuna).

The Tantrist knows that two physiologically crucial moments occur in every human life, and the possibility of a third such moment exists for the "thrice-blessed" woman.

Orgasm is the first such experience, and all that is required to transmute the physical sensations into another dimension is the mutual concentration of both parties upon an appropriate God-image of each other, accompanied by mantric invocation. Even this can be dispensed with if the attitude toward each other's body is profound worship (in Old English, spelled "worthship"), based on the knowledge that the physical temple is truly "worthy" of adoration.

There are two points to consider. The first is that Tantra as well as Western Esoteric practice sees Divinity in every man and every woman. To confine ourselves for the moment to those raised in a Judeo-Christian environment, for one to say that "we are created in God's image" is to assert that there is indeed a "spark of Divinity" at the core of every person. The second concerns the goal of all ritual, whether very simple or very complex, *which is to exalt the Divine Spark.* This is the key formula to the transformation of the person, for to exalt the inner Divinity will lead the person into Divinity.

To see God/Goddess as incarnate in the person of your beloved, and to experience oneself as God/Goddess both in your inner essence as well as in the eyes of your lover is truly powerful magick!

Although not mentioned in classical texts, it is obvious that childbirth is another such peak period. One who determines to retain awareness at the exact moment of the emergence of her child into the stream of life may be caught up into a never-before-experienced consciousness of the universal and eternal.

The last of these automatic opportunities for higher

consciousness may be manifested at death by an individual who strives to die in a conscious manner, with his mind seeking attainment of a superconscious state. This science of "passing over" is highly developed among Tibetan Tantrists who aid the process by pressing upon certain nerve centers and pressure points in the neck of the dying monk.

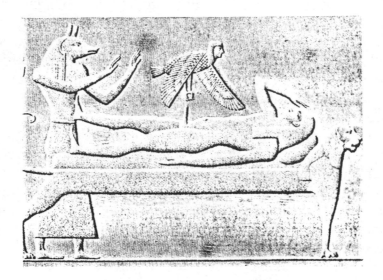

These three experiences all involve altered physiological activity of the body, accompanied by corresponding psychological changes. The Tantric procedure in each case is to ride the crest of emotion and, at the apogee of the experience, thrust the mind higher through an appropriate concentrative method. The result sought is the transcendental bliss, or Samadhi, of the Yogi.

Tantra utilizes basic sexual excitation to flood the brain with sensations so strong that extraneous mental activity is obliterated or pushed out of the field of consciousness. Patanjali's definition, "Yoga is the cessation of the fluctuations of the mind-stuff," becomes a psychophysical reality, for at the instant of convulsive spasm, consciousness of "doing" ceases and consciousness of "BEING" reigns. Orgasm is the only spontaneous, natural experience of a deathless, birthless, timeless, sorrowless dimension.

Tantra is the way of the Hero (Vira) who neither rejects nor fears any aspect of life. The Tantrist seeks freedom (Moksha) through life (sensation, sentient, sensual) and not through escape (abstinence, abstaining, absence), using the body as an instrument of evolution. In the words of a Tantric proverb, "He who would rise must first thrust himself up with the aid of the earth."

Tantra is the science of the Earth-mother, substituting feeling for logic, sensation for cerebration, and active touching for passive viewing.

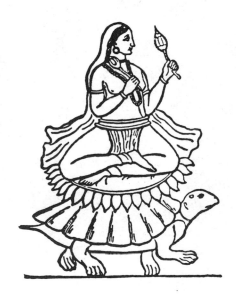

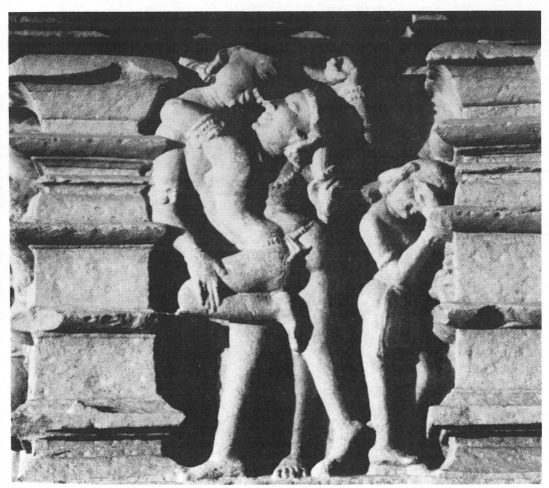

Lakshmana Temple, Khajuraho.

Psychosexual Power and Tantric Exercises

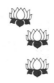

TO EXPERIENCE TANTRIC ecstasy, the psyche must first be freed of negative attitudes toward sex and have achieved a basic sexual awareness. Several flat statements are required in discussing the psychic aspects of sexuality. The sexual experience is dependent upon integration of the nervous system. If one considers the achievement of orgasm as analogous to launching a rocket to hit the moon (i.e., a climax), then it is an unequivocal fact that so far as the neural pathways in the nervous system are concerned, the method by which the sexual skyrocket is launched is of absolutely no consequence. All the nervous system is concerned with is that contact explosion in inner space. The firing modality, be it masturbation, homosexuality, or heterosexuality, is irrelevant. Theoretically, only the end result (orgasm) is important, and any form of sexual behavior is but a means to an end: the cessation of fluctuations of mind, producing timeless transcendence.

When it comes to practice, of course, we find our

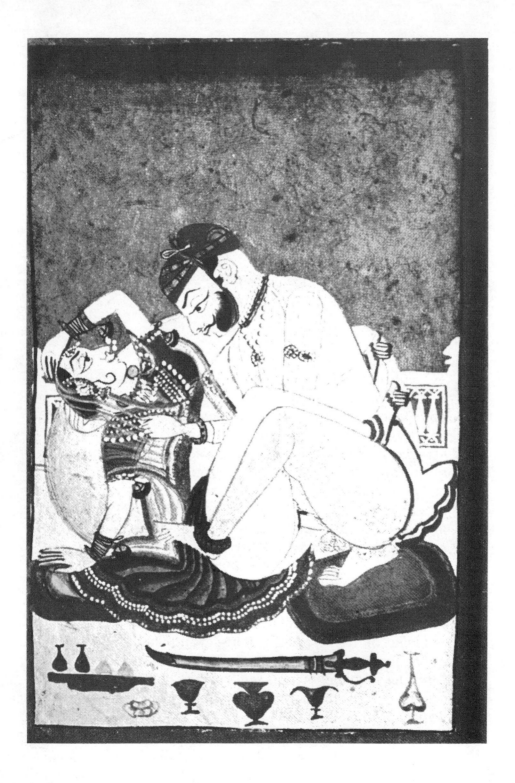

ability to achieve orgasm limited by attitude, the intervening variable between genital and brain. Only attitude, a product of social conditioning, prevents many from exploring their inherent bisexual nature or fully reaping the psychic benefits of autoeroticism and heterosexual copulation.

In the latter half of the twentieth century we intellectually know that most sexual prejudices are irrational but we may continue to react emotionally to some possibilities of sexual variation. Psychologists are rewriting textbooks in view of the fact that a concept of sexual deviation or abnormality is no longer tenable. In ancient China and India the concept that some forms of sexual behavior were abnormal was virtually nonexistent. The idea of "sexual crime" is limited strictly to those cases that interfere with the free will of another person, e.g., rape.

Just as one can talk about physics or metaphysics, so one can talk about sex or "metasex" (a term introduced by Marco Vassi in his *Penthouse* article, "The Eroticum"). When I use the neologism "metasex," I am implying that sexual activity in a human being is multidimensional. We can look at sex from a number of different levels. The primal level is "procreational sex." Procreational sex perpetuates the species, and we exist by virtue of this dimension. As Aleister Crowley pointed out in his *Eight Lectures on Yoga*, that yoking of an ovum and spermatozoa is the first great Yoga or union. It is the most marvelous of all Yogas because no one knows what potential genius will arise out of that linking. Beyond the procreational mode, we enter the realm of what some zoologists would call "recreational sex"—sex for play, relaxation, and the combating of boredom.

"Tranquilizing sex" is yet another dimension. Sexual activity in human beings can and should be used as a natural tranquilizer. This form offers an inexhaustible supply of built-in Valium or Librium tablets with few side-effects. A simple example of tranquilizing sex is the use of masturbation to cure insomnia; freeing the mind-body

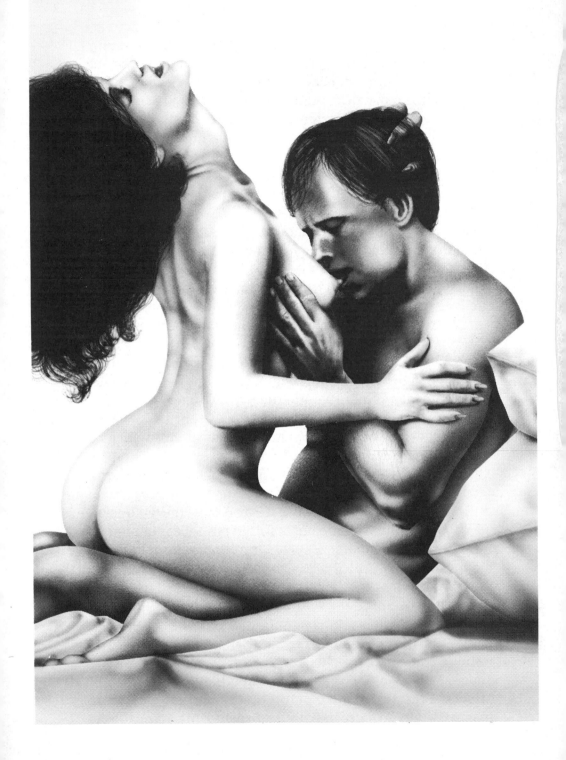

complex of tension, it permits sleep. Unfortunately, most of us have been subjected to various types of guilt-conditioning which can interfere with our ability to utilize sex as the most natural of tranquilizing and curative agents.

Many people, because of tension and negative conditioning, will only permit themselves a sexual experience when absolutely everything else is correct in both the external and internal environments. In other words, everything has to be right: no headaches, no stomach aches, no cramps, no emotional turmoil, and then maybe they will go and relax in a special room and have something they call "sex." The problem is that very seldom on any given day is everything just right or "perfect."

The *occult* approach to sexuality is that one doesn't wait for the right circumstances to have some sort of internal erotic experience—rather one goes ahead and has a sexual experience to readjust the psychic equilibrium of the nervous system and thus *make* things go right.

Some occultists misuse sexuality for the purposes of "black magic." In fact, sexuality is a specific antidote, as well as antithesis, to "black magic." The deliberate trying (and "try" is a word with built-in failure) to injure another person, mentally or physically, through psychic channels is only resorted to by those who are psychologically ill and feel themselves to be impotent in negotiating life. Paranoid personalities, riddled with feelings of envy, hostility, suspiciousness and oversensitivity, characterize those prone to practice "black magic," and these very traits trip them up because they are susceptible to the idea that their own spells will rebound upon them. "Black magic" is a type of mental judo in which an attempt is made to surface the victim's innate, and normally unconscious, negativity and fear, turning it against him while simultaneously convincing him that the force is external to himself.

Psychological maturity confers immunity to "black magic." Depth psychotherapy—Freudian, Jungian or Reichian—is the best single prophylactic and cure against exposure to noxious aspects of occultism.

The notion that sexuality can be used to achieve destructive objectives is as restrictive and debilitating to occultists as traditional sexual prejudices are to the population at large. Sex magic is not an appropriate vehicle for "black magic" because the psychic projectile of charged hate and anger is the antithesis of the emotional states generating an orgasm. In fact, sexual sorcery is an excellent expedient for strengthening a shattered psyche or pulling together a sick ego. Esoteric psychology teaches that the powerful force fields created by mutual orgasm repair lesions in the auric shields of the male and female by virtue of the intensity of "re-pairing."

Tantric sexuality is the dimension of sex employed for *consciousness expansion.* One possible translation of the Sanskrit prefix *tan* is "expand," while *tra* means "liberate"; so Tantra becomes that which first "expands" and then "liberates" the mind. A colloquial translation of Tantra would be "mind-blowing."

In terms of profound sexual experience, this consciousness expansion is produced by the far-reaching effects that tactile or touch receptors exert upon brain states and personality. We even describe personality idiosyncrasies using such tactile synonyms as "touchy," "prickly," "smooth," "rough" and "silky" or "soft." The importance of adequate tactile stimulation in character development is driven home by our reference to a person who is consistently thoughtless, insensitive to the feelings of others and verbally callous as "tact-less." *Sexual experience is primarily touch or tactile sensation.*

Standard psychophysiological estimates of daily sensory

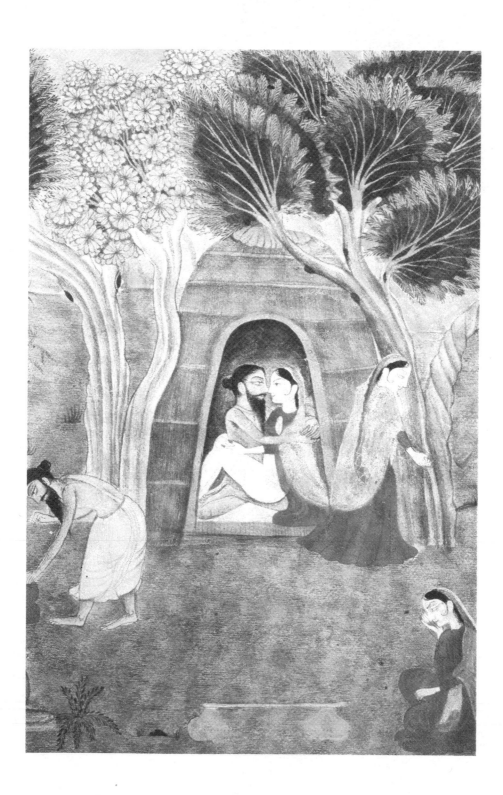

information input to the brain reveal the following per-
centages: 75 percent information via sight; 13 percent
information via hearing; 6 percent information via smell
and taste; 6 percent information via touch. Although only
6 percent of our total environmental information comes to
us through tactile nerve endings, it has been recognized
for thousands of years in Asia that it is not *quantity* but
quality that is important. The most exquisite sensory sensation that man is capable of having comes through the
tactile receptors that give rise to orgasm. The climax is the
ultimate tactile sensation, the tactile sensation that ideally
eradicates tension, blows the mind, induces consciousness
expansion and leaves an aftermath of lucidity.

The path to psychosexual power begins not only with
recognizing and overcoming restrictive sexual prejudices,
but also with cultivating intense gonadal awareness through
conscious tightening of the pelvic floor. This is accomplished
through deliberate, selective contraction and relaxation of
the anal and urethral (urinary) sphincters.

These exercises have been traditional for thousands
of years in Tantra Yoga and throughout the Middle East.
The techniques have recently been rediscovered by
Western gynecologists and sex therapists such as Dr. Kegal
and Drs. Masters and Johnson. We should remember that
the word "discover" etymologically means to "uncover,"
so in actuality there is "nothing new under the sun." The
encounter movement in psychology still has much to
rediscover or "uncover" from Tantra in regard to touch
therapy.

EXERCISE ONE: *MULA BANDHA*
This is a perineum or pelvic contraction lock which
begins at the anal sphincter and spreads forward to the
genitals. KEY: the correct feeling of anal locking may be
understood by recalling the sensation induced by holding

back the passage of stool from the bowel or retaining an enema.

METHOD:

- *Step One:* Sit erect in any comfortable position, hands palm up on the thighs.

- *Step Two:* Focus attention on the anal region, beginning with awareness of the floor or chair exerting pressure up against the buttocks and then pinpoint consciousness upon the anus.

- *Step Three:* Inhale a half-lungful of air, swallow and retain breath.

- *Step Four:* Slowly contract the anus to maximum while continuing to hold the breath. N. B. Breath is retained throughout up to step six.

- *Step Five: Women:* spread pelvic floor contraction forward from the anus until a distinct twitch is felt in the vaginal lips. *Men:* spread pelvic floor contraction forward from the anus until a distinct pull is felt upon testicles resting in scrotal sac.

- *Step Six:* Release pelvic contraction completely, take in a sniff of fresh air and then smoothly exhale fully.

Advantages of Mula Bandha:

- Tones the anal sphincters, preventing and curing (in early stages) hemorrhoids and anal pruritus.

- Sends a blood flush stimulating the uro-genital system in both men and women.

- *Women:* tightens slack vaginal walls and reduces tendency toward so-called frigidity or orgasmic impairment; *Men:* reduces tendency for premature ejaculation and impotence.

- Awakens Muladhara Chakra.

EXERCISE TWO: *VAJROLI MUDRA*

This is a simplified form of the classical Vajroli Mudra revealed to the Western world by the greatest living exponent of the nonsexual aspects of Tantra, Swami Parahansa Satyananda Saraswati of Monghyr, India. KEY: Vajroli Mudra involves urethral sphincter closure exactly as when you cut off the flow of urine in midstream while voiding.

Preliminary awareness training: Drink several pints of water on an empty stomach. In an hour, empty the bladder. Practice cutting off and restarting the urine flow at least a dozen times until the bladder is fully drained.

METHOD:

- *Step One:* Sit erect in any comfortable position, hands palm up on the thighs.

- *Step Two:* Focus attention on the urethral sphincter, below the clitoris in women and at the base of the penis (near the pubic bone) in men.

- *Step Three:* Inhale a half-lungful of air, swallow and retain the breath.

- *Step Four:* Contract urethral orifice exactly as when cutting off urine flow and at the same time pull up the lower abdomen as if attempting to suck genitals into the pelvis. Relax the contraction and repeat as many times as possible on that breath, allowing a feeling of sexual excitement to spread up the spinal cord from the pelvis to the brain.

- *Step Five:* Cease the contractions, relax the abdomen, take in a sniff of fresh air and then smoothly exhale fully.

Auxiliary check exercise: *Women:* gently insert one or two fingers in the vagina and perform Vajroli Mudra. When done correctly contractions should spread, causing the vagina to clasp the fingers gently. *Men:* perform Vajroli

Mudra standing naked in front of the mirror. Watch to check that the head of the penis twitches or elevates slightly with each contraction.

Advantages of Vajroli Mudra:

- Tones urethral sphincter, preventing and curing (in early stages) urinary stress incontinence.

- Sends blood flush stimulating uro-genital system in both men and women.

- *Women:* encourages clitoral sensitivity. *Men:* encourages erectile potency.

- Awakens Swadhisthana Chakra.

Mula Bandha should be followed by Vajroli Mudra daily, beginning with ten repetitions of each, adding five additional repetitions a week until a maximum of sixty rounds each is performed a day. One round equals completion from the first step to last. Note that some people will achieve better control with three-quarters of a lungful of air or even full lungs rather than with the suggested half-breath. The sniff of air in the final step of each exercise is a Pranayama device designed by Gurudev Satyananda of Bihar Yoga school to give instant relief after Kumbhaka (breath retention) and permit a controlled, full exhalation.

Mula Bandha and Vajroli Mudra develop pelvic thrust ability in the male and penile gripping power in the female, enhancing sensitivity and control during intercourse for both sexes.

Intercourse, from French and Latin, was formerly *entercourse*. The Tantric sexual embrace allows each partner to *enter a course* into the astral unconscious realms of the mind, facilitating the building between (inter) Shiva and Shakti of a bridge (course) or psychic channel.

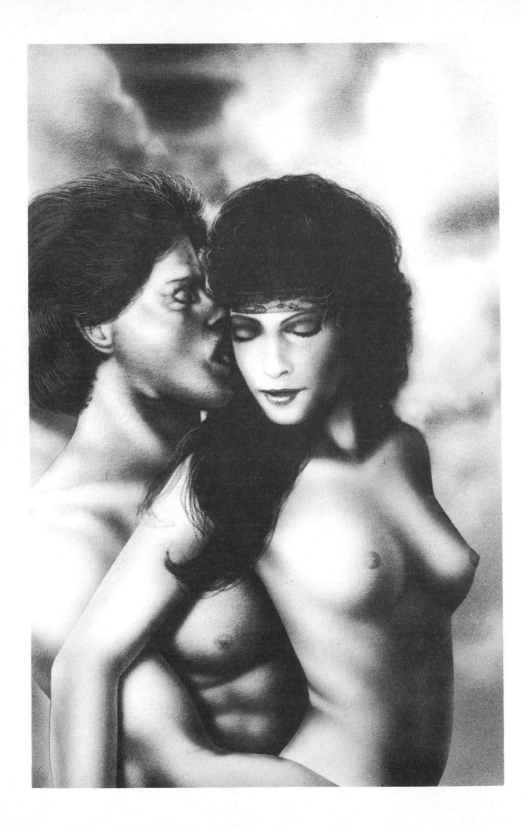

Asanas of Love *for* *Kundalini Arousal*

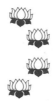

WITHIN THE CONTEXT of this manual a fundamental difference exists between sex magic and Tantra. Sex magic may be employed, unaccompanied by emotional commitment to the partner, in order to change one's attitudes or favorably influence a situation. Simple concentration upon the desired goal, in the form of an image, while experiencing climax, inevitably brings a result. Sex magic is the most powerful form of self-hypnosis known.

Tantra, however, is designed to alter (through worshiping another's body altar) the state of consciousness of the participants and generally requires that the fire of emotion—designated love—be concomitant with sexual excitement.

Tantra teaches that the total sexual experience may be a path to freedom (Moksha), dissolving the ego (Ahamkara). Ritual intercourse is a tool for consciousness expansion, overwhelming the incessant chatter of the thinking brain (cerebral cortex) with a flood of orgasmic excitement triggered by sensations

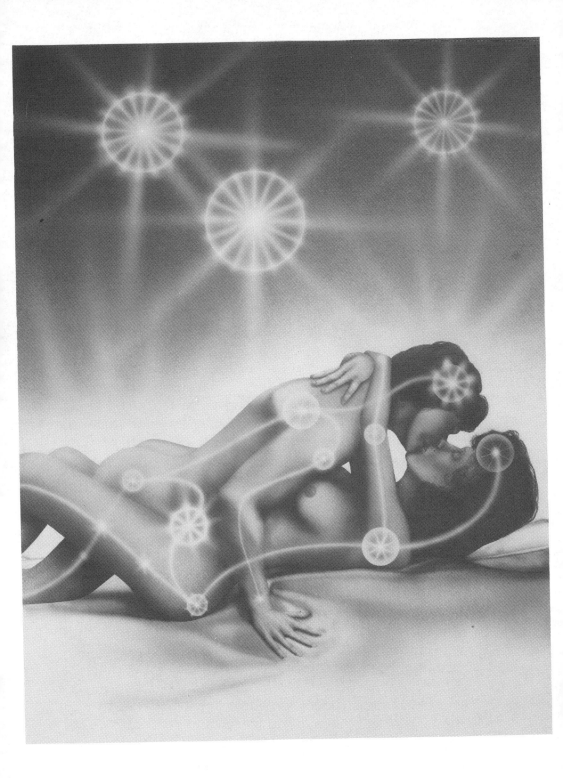

in the erogenous zones. Body energies are used for cosmic bliss, with the understanding that there is a difference between "using" and "being used." "Use" not "ab-use" is the key.

Touch and tactile stimulus are so closely related to emotions that we not only use the word "feel" to describe both texture and emotion, but even employ the word "touch" to convey emotion, as in the expression "I was touched by your poetry." Emotion tends, and is intended, to translate itself into action so that it is colloquially expressed in such terms as "I was deeply moved . . ."
The Tantric orgasm instantly produces:

- Cessation of fluctuations of the mind ("Yoga is the cessation of the fluctuations of the mind stuff." Patanjali Yoga Sutras, Book 1, Verse 2, c. 200 B.C.).

- Freedom from the past and future, suspending consciousness in point-instant time.

- Opening of the psychic centers in the head (Ajna Chakra and Sahasrara Chakra) resulting in psychedelic visions.

The Panch Tattwas or Panch Makaras is a basic Tantric ritual of the "five good things" which has captivated the imagination of Westerners. This rite is the partaking of wine (Madya), meat (Mamsa), fish (Matsya), parched grain (Mudra) and intercourse (Maithuna). These five things have several different levels of interpretation, and many commentators on Tantra—Eastern and Western—have pretended that the ceremony is only an allegory.

At a literal level, the reader will perceive that an orthodox vegetarian and abstemious Hindu would shake himself loose from his cultural roots, "blowing" his mind by imbibing forbidden wine, meat, fish, and indulging in copulation under circumstances devoid of the usual ritual prerequisites and

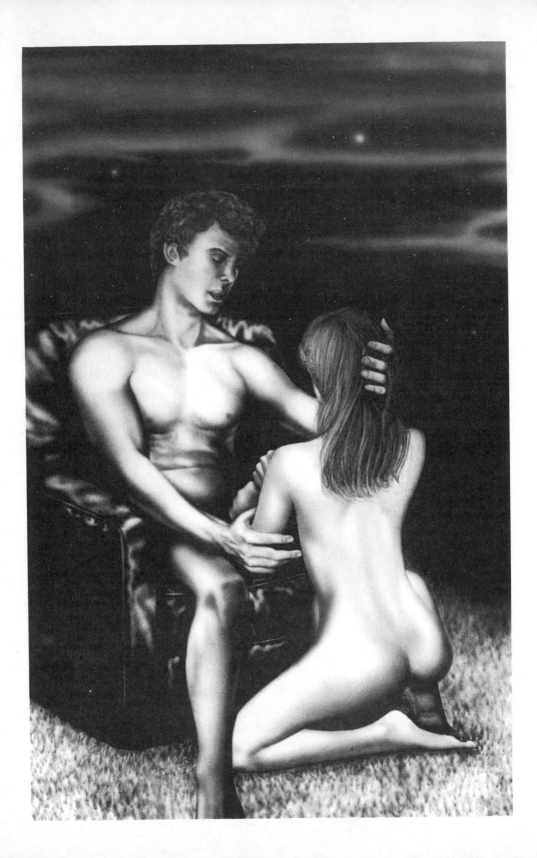

taboos. In this sense, *Tantra is an organized system which rejects nothing as a means to a spiritual end.* It takes advantage of shock tactics to catapult the mind into a transcendent state beyond normal social and caste restrictions. The Panch Makaras are designed to induce delirium, madness and ecstasy.

Another level of interpretation reveals the "five good things" as sexual variations leading to a crescendo of orgasmic experience. In one system the wine is composed of saliva, vaginal secretions and semen. The meat eaten is the fellatio, or oral intercourse performed by the female partner, Shakti, upon the Lingam of her Lord Shiva. The fish is cunnilingus, in which Shiva worships the Yoni of his Shakti with his tongue, feeling her as a living embodiment of the Castle of Brahman. The parched grain is the position or posture (Asana) undertaken by both male and female for intercourse, in which the fire upon the genital altar is created by the friction of the Lingam and Yoni, exquisitely brushing each other, much as two sticks rubbed together will heat and ignite. The actual intercourse becomes an enactment of Vedic sacrifice in which pure ghee or butter (semen) is poured into the fire upon the altar (vagina).

ORAL CONGRESS *(AUPARISHTAKA)*

The uniting of mouth and genitals frustrates the normal procreation-oriented flow of sexual energies and produces a psychic short-circuit which quickly arouses Kundalini, inducing spiritual rapture and immobilizing thought.

The intimate connection between the mouth and the sexual organs is concealed in such sayings as "She's a real dish," "You look good enough to eat," "A luscious figure," and the current English euphemism for cunnilingus: "He eats me."

The importance of oral sex in adulthood is not mysterious, considering that the infant's first experience of

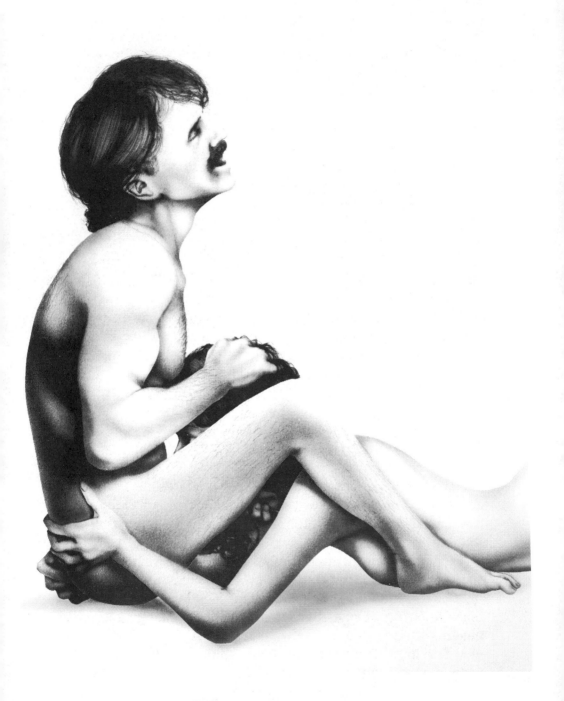

pleasure and comfort comes from suckling the breast to relieve the tension of hunger. Thereafter, the mouth is a source of comfort, so the weaned child sucks its thumb when nervous and, during the first years of school, instinctively chews on the end of a pencil when anxiously concentrating. The early adolescent seeks oral gratification with gum and quickly graduates to cigarettes, pipes and cigars as an adult.

Tantra and sex magic recognize fellatio and cunnilingus as a yoga integrating consciousness by joining polar opposites. That which is above affixes to that which is below—following the Hermetic (the word implies a "seal") axiom, "As above, so below"—to create mental children rather than physical progeny. The exoteric act of depositing semen within the vagina means that the physical and psychic properties of sperm are utilized to perpetuate the race physically, thus ensuring survival of the species.

Vajroli Mudra, fellatio and cunnilingus redirect psychic

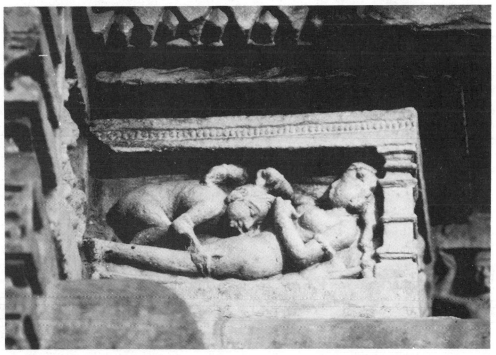

Cunnilingus, Lakshmana Temple, Khajuraho.

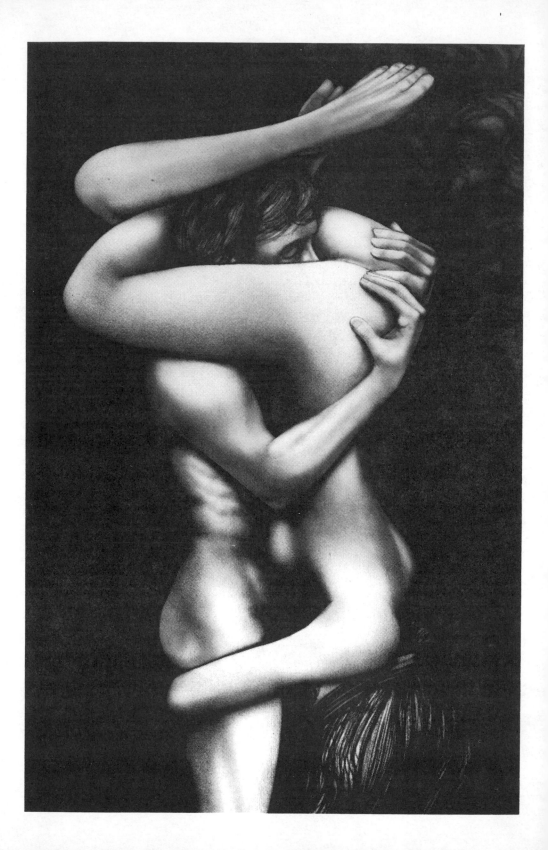

forces so that a "brainchild"—i.e., an idea or "concept"—is magically conceived. Such a "brainchild" is immortal, out-living any mere physical, finite span of existence that could be achieved through physical birth.

"Cunni-lingus" substitutes the phallic tongue for the penis, while fellatio replaces the vagina with the mouth. The result in both cases is a "mind explosion." The yogic practice of linking mouth and tongue with the genital com-plex bombards the brain with an eruption of sexual, tactile impulses which unfold the Dalas, or petals, of each psy-chic center.

The famous "Descartes illusion" is testimony to the hypersensitivity of the tongue when applied to the clitoris or head of the penis. The French philosopher Rene Descartes (1596–1650) noted the tongue as a tactile magnifier par excellence. He observed how a tooth cavity the size of a pinhead feels as large as a matchhead when touched with the tip of the tongue. This capacity of the tongue to pro-duce such a perceptual illusion of enlargement forms the basis for the effective employment of oral sex in Tantric ritual.

The ability of the mouth to produce saliva is a reflec-tion of our emotional or psychic state. Fear leaves the mouth dry and parched; hence our custom of placing a glass of water on the lecture platform in anticipation of nervous speakers. Conversely, when we are sexually excited during oral congress, the mouth floods with saliva, providing the philosopher's tincture with which the alchemical genital secretions may be mixed to form an elixir. It should be noted that the vagina, like the mouth, parches with fear or floods with ecstasy.

Any repugnance to oral sex among Westerners is due to widespread confusion about the difference between bodily excretions (waste products no longer needed) and sexual secretions (fluids rich in nutrients). Perfect genital hygiene is a prerequisite to Tantra, and it must be emphasized that however lacking in concern about public sanitation Easterners appear to be, their personal hygiene is immaculate.

In Yoga the terminals for releasing Pranic energies are the hands and feet. Tantric doctrine views the tongue and the genital area as the great radiators or throw-off points for subtle forces. Thus, the use of fellatio and cunnilingus in sex magic releases immense reserves of psychic force to sweep vigorously through the nervous system; the traditional "battery terminals" connect, closing the circuit for bioenergies to be exchanged between two practitioners.

The association between mouth and genitalia is suggested in the folklore that the impassioned Goddess who involuntarily parts her lips in ecstasy is ripe to spread her thighs, parting the labia or genital lips. "As above, so below."

ORAL INTERCOURSE POSTURE (KAKISANA*)

The male (Shakta) and female (Shakti) lie on their right sides facing so that the head of each partner is opposite the genital region of the other. The man slips his right hand underneath the thighs of the woman, cradling his head between her thighs. Moistening his right thumb and index finger with saliva, he seals her anus firmly with the pad of his index finger while gently inserting the thumb (nail pared, smooth and clean) into the vagina. He applies his mouth and tongue to the Yoni, favoring her clitoris. The Goddess (Devi) encapsulates his Lingam with her mouth, locking the urethral orifice with the tongue and pressing his anus with the third finger, using the remaining fingers and thumb of her right hand to caress his perineum and scrotum. Mutual orgasm is brought about as slowly as possible, allowing the consciousness of Radha and Krishna to freeze into transcendent immobility.

---

*"The Crow Posture." The Sanskrit terms used for Tantric sexual embraces are often similar to those used in Hatha Yoga but seldom have any resemblance to the Hatha Asana of the same name.

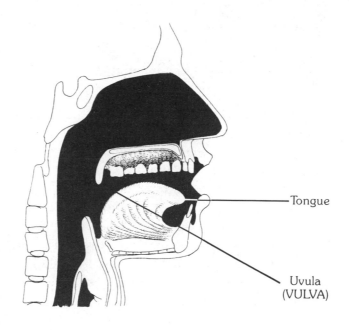

Tongue

Uvula
(VULVA)

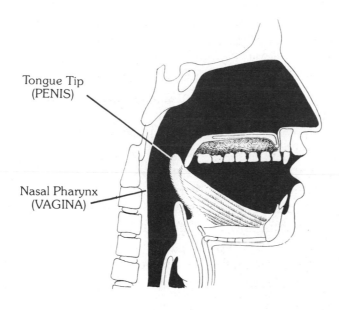

Tongue Tip
(PENIS)

Nasal Pharynx
(VAGINA)

**Sexual Symbolism of
Khechari Mudra**

THE AUTOSEXUAL GESTURE
(KHECHARI MUDRA)

Khechari Mudra is an advanced Hatha Yoga and Tantric technique in which the tongue is seemingly swallowed. In actual fact, the tip of the tongue is thrust deep into the nasal-pharynx region behind and above the soft palate.

This is accomplished by the adept's stretching the tongue daily and gradually wearing away the fraenum linguae (fold of mucous membrane tying the tongue to the floor of the mouth) across the front incisor teeth.*

The psychophysiological results of this action are profound, which is hardly surprising when we realize the importance of the tongue as an organ indispensably necessary in the four distinct functions of speech (articulation), chewing (mastication), tasting (gustation), and swallowing (deglutition).

The neural connections of the autonomic and central nervous systems to the tongue are profuse. This is evidenced by the involvement of five of the twelve pair of cranial nerves with the tongue. The cranial nerves emerge from the base of the brain and the upper bulb of the spinal cord.

The five cranial nerves are: the trigeminal nerve (fifth cranial), conveying sensations of pain, heat, cold and touch from the tongue to the brain; the facial nerve (seventh cranial), carrying taste from the front two-thirds of the tongue; the glosso-pharyngeal nerve (ninth cranial), transmitting taste from the posterior or back third of the tongue; the vagus nerve (tenth cranial), responsible for taste fibers located on the epiglottis and arytenoid cartilages of the voice box (the vagus also governs swallowing actions of the tongue); the hypoglossal nerve (twelfth cranial), mastering all muscular movements of the tongue.

Indian research studies published in the *Yoga Mimamsa Journal* (Vol. XII, No. 2, October, 1969) indicate that Khechari Mudra lowers the body basal metabolic rate

---

*Some people are able to do this without previous stretching, or cutting, of the fraenum linguae.

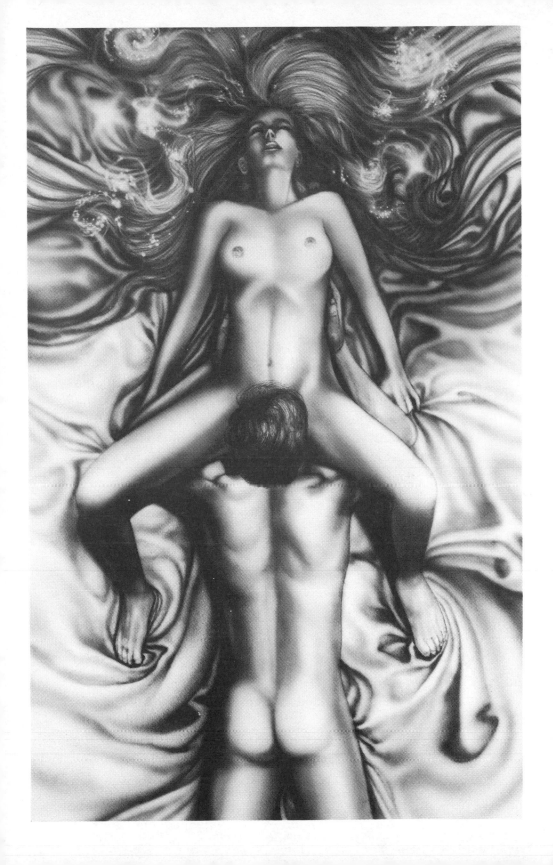

(BMR), or oxygen consumption, by twenty-five percent, with no decrease in energy level. The subject used in this study had practiced Khechari about three years. During 1970 I gave several public demonstrations of Kumbhaka (Yoga breath retention) in the five-minute range without prior hyperventilation. My mastery of Khechari Mudra made such feats virtually effortless.

Some Tantric systems consider Khechari Mudra to be Mamsa, i.e., eating the meat of the Panch Makaras ritual. The word "Khechari" means "wandering in space," implying the exploration of inner or mental space.

From the viewpoint of occult anatomy, the tongue is the penis of the mouth, the nasal-pharynx is the vagina, and the "u"-shaped fleshy portion of the soft palate called the uvula (by Temurah,* the "Vulva") is the clitoris.

Khechari Mudra traps positive and negative psychic forces in the head, through the symbolic penetration of the phallic tongue into the vaginal naso-pharynx. This gesture unites Shakti and Shakta, Kundalini and Shiva, Radha and Krishna, the Lingam (intellectual nature) and Yoni (emotional nature) of the psychological microcosm.

Khechari Mudra is the sign of autosexual intercourse with the self, signaling an ultimate, secret message to the unconscious of eternity. It is the serpent swallowing his own tail.

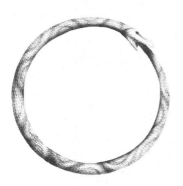

In the words of the Hatha-Yoga Pradipika, "When one has closed the hole at the root of the palate through the Khechari Mudra his seminal fluid is not emitted even though he is embraced by a young and passionate woman."

*See Chapter 6.

ANAL INTERCOURSE* (ADHORATA)

Anal intercourse is the Tantric equivalent of such Hatha Yoga practices as Mulabandha (anal sphincter lock), and Asvini Mudra (alternating relaxation and contraction of the anus).

The secret tradition of magical Tantra teaches that the anus is an ultrasensitive erogenic and psychic zone directly linked to Muladhara, the basal Chakra. Hidden within Muladhara, coiled and compressed like a spring, lies the primal power of the nervous system manifest as the Snake Goddess, Kundalini.

The anatomical essence of a human being is the thirty-two feet of continuous hollow tube, extending from mouth to anus, known as the gastrointestinal tract.

In Lawrence Durrell's *Justine,* Balthazar, the cabalistic physician, comments, "After all the work of philosophers on his soul and the doctors on his body, what can we say we really know about man? That he is, when all is said and done, just a passage for liquids and solids, A PIPE OF FLESH."

The terminus for the "pipe of flesh" is the anus, composed of an internal and external sphincter, rings of muscle surrounding a body orifice. The word "sphincter" means a "knot" or a "band" and is derived from the same Greek base as "Sphinx," the mythological beast epitomizing occult mysteries. The master of Tantric sex magic opens the anal sphincters of his Shakti, thus solving the riddle of the Sphinx.

Anal intercourse is a specific Kundalini arousal method. Reference to *Gray's Anatomy* reveals the existence of an irregular, oval-shaped gland between the rectal wall and the tip of the tailbone, or coccyx, called the "coccygeal body." Although the function of this gland is unknown to

---

* Anal intercourse is not encouraged as part of a Tantric regimen during the current AIDS crisis. Even with the use of a condom, too little is understood about the transmission of the virus to risk the disease.

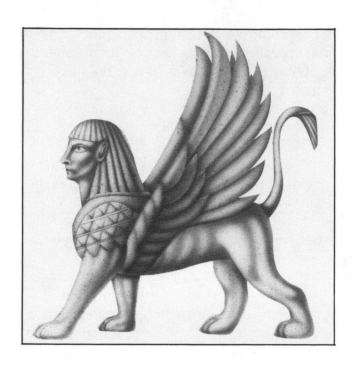

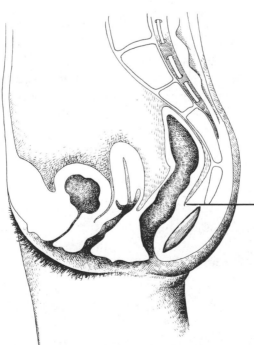

Kundalini Gland

Western physiologists, it is established in Tantra as the "Kundalini gland." Yoga has devised a wide variety of techniques to irritate and awaken this gland into activity, including Mula Bandha, Asvini Mudra, Tada Mudra (knocking the buttocks upon the ground, sending rhythmic shock waves rippling up the spine), and rolling on a cotton ball placed under the tip of the tailbone.

Tantric activation of the gland is direct and swift through the dilation of the anal sphincters, with a consequent reflex effect upon the two branches of the autonomic nervous system. These two branches, terminating in the anus and rectum, are the parasympathetic (Ida, or braking influence) and the sympathetic (Pingala, or accelerating influence). As well as altering the state of the involuntary nervous system, anal intercourse, according to traditional belief, results in the ejaculation of semen into the rectum, which nourishes the "Kundalini gland" much as the white of an egg feeds the fertilized yolk or embryo. The Tantrist, sustaining his Shakti or Goddess with anal intercourse, facilitates the arousal of her internal fire.

The Occidental mentality is conditioned to look upon the anus as unclean. The Hindu, on the other hand, is scrupulous in hygiene at both ends of the "pipe of flesh," having a firm tradition of rinsing the anus after bowel activity, using copious quantities of water and the left hand (the right hand being reserved for handling food when eating!). Certain schools of Hatha Yoga consider washing the bowel daily with water through a system of natural enemas (Basti) as much a necessity as cleaning the mouth and teeth.

Common sense dictates avoidance of vaginal intercourse after anal intercourse because bacteria comfortably established in the colon could be transferred to the foreign environment of the vagina, causing bladder infections.

Tantric practices may be viewed by some as "pervert" or "deviate," and in terms of the inner meaning of these words, they are. "Pervert" means "to overthrow," "to turn around," while "deviate" (*de* and *via*, the way or path) suggests "off the road," "out of the way."

Tantric sexual methodology induces a psychic short-circuit. Webster defines a short circuit as: "A new pathway made by a current where it encounters a smaller resistance than in the normal circuit, thus allowing a much larger current to flow through and causing dangerous overheating or fusing." "Dangerous overheating" in a psychic sense includes neurotic guilt reactions, while "fusing" implies fusion of the mind-body complex.

Tantra uses anal intercourse as a sexual variation to potentiate internal processes leading to heightened consciousness.

AWAKENING THE CHAKRAS THROUGH INTERCOURSE

Tantric Maithuna is an exercise in sensory awareness. If one focuses attention on the correct sensory avenue during love-making, the specific chakra corresponding to that sensation will blossom. A chakra is a whirling vortex of energy at the conjunction point of mind and body. Anatomically, the chakras correspond to ductless glands and major plexuses of the autonomic or involuntary nervous system.

The first five psychic centers are opened by calling into play their associated sensory gates. Ajna, the sixth center, and Sahasrara, the seventh, open automatically, depending on the intensity of the climax.

The effectiveness of Tantra as a psychosexual event stimulating the subtle body and its inherent force centers is dependent upon prolonging the psychic tension leading to orgasm. Westerners are too anxious for mutual, explosive relief bringing the sexual experience to a quick end. The Tantrist concentrates upon the "means" rather than the "end," *thus maintaining a special preclimactic state as*

SAHASRARA

AJNA

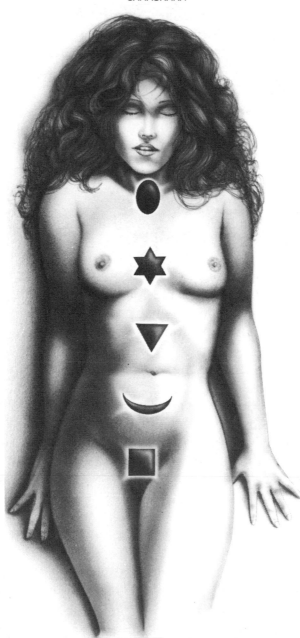

VISHUDDHI
Pharyngeal Plexus,
Thyroid and Parathy-
roids.

ANAHATA
Cardio-pulmonary
Plexus, Thymus

MANIPURA
Solar Plexus,
Pancreas

SWADHISTHANA
Hyprogastric Plexus,
Suprarenal Glands

MULADHARA
Pelvic Plexus, Ovaries
and Testes

SOUND: heartbeat,
breathing, digestive
gurglings, cries of
ecstasy, sucking
sound of the
convulsive vagina.

TOUCH: caressing,
tactile impulses from
the clitoris, penis
and tongue.

SIGHT: adoration of
partner's body, while
motionless, allowing
psychic tension to
build.

TASTE: saltiness of
skin, saliva, fresh
genital secretions
produced in a state
of excitement.

SMELL: perfume,
incense, fresh
perspiration and
natural genital odors
produced in a state
of excitement.

Tantric sensory routes to the Chakras

long as possible. The Sanskrit "Tantra" (to weave, extend, stretch) is related to the Latin *tendere* (to stretch, strain), giving rise to a host of associated concepts such as attenuate, tension, tone, tendon, tend and tender (to reach out, offer). Tantra is the attending, with tenderness, to another's psychophysiological being, while building the fire of sexual-emotional tension. The result extends and attenuates the consciousness until—like an overstretched rubber band—the mind snaps, temporarily disintegrating the ego, or "little self."

TANTRIC INTERCOURSE POSTURES

The postures illustrated on the following pages, despite their variations, embody a number of unique features. The Yoga of penis and vagina is achieved with the female (Shakti) in an upright position sitting astride the male and facing him. The erect posture of both participants in the Tantric Eucharist adds a new dimension of intensified orgasm and positive affirmation to sexual experience.

In Hindu Tantra, the woman is power personified and as such is always active, the Lingam moving in her Yoni like a pestle grinding inside an inverted mortar. She has reversed the normal social and psychological roles of male and female, transforming herself into the active, dominant force milking the penis of virile energies.

The sitting-up posture ("sitting-down" postures are considered nonexistent in Yoga) firmly locks the Lingam (penis) in the Yoni (vagina), preventing it from slipping out, even after ejaculation.

The tendency of the semen, pulled down by gravity, is to drain away from the mouth of the uterus, thus confirming Tantric intercourse as a magical and psychic, rather than procreative, act.

While embracing, both parties can simultaneously

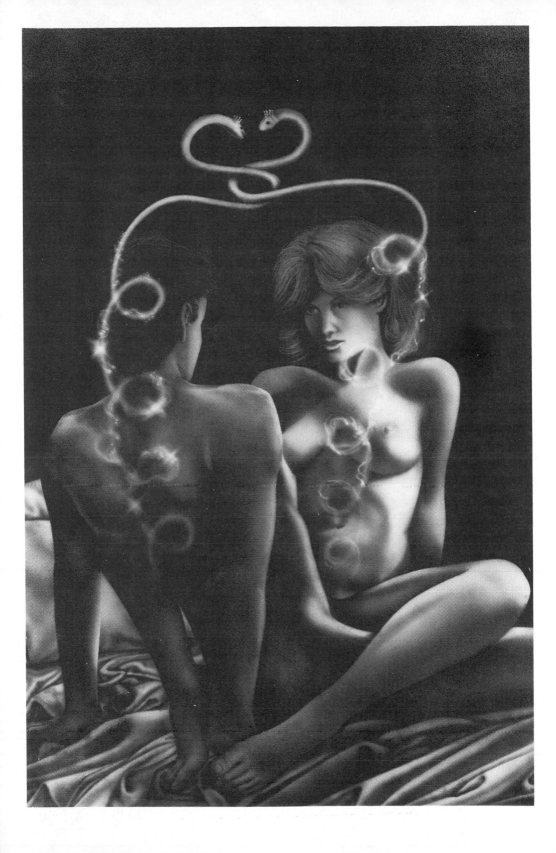

engage in a gentle rocking and swaying to-and-fro movement which powerfully relaxes the nervous system. The efficacy of this movement is probably due to an awakening of unconscious memories of free-floating in the amniotic waters of the womb; the movement is similar to the rocking infants indulge in.

In all of these postures, the ideal is to achieve virtually simultaneous orgasms for the most powerful sex magic and Kundalini arousal. Direct clitoral stimulation of the female is favored by these positions.

I have arranged the Maithuna Asanas in order, according to suppleness required. Only the first two necessitate the Padmasana or full-lotus posture by the male. Those lacking a mastery of the lotus may be assured that psychic results are just as strong in the easier variations, for it is the concentration that is important.(See color plates after page 76.)

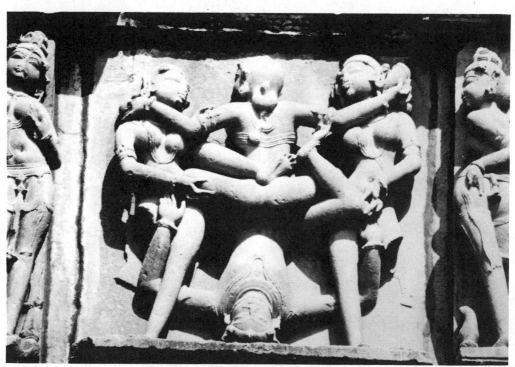

Kandariya Mahadeva Temple, Khajuraho

A Tantric Synoptic Commentary on the Shat Chakras

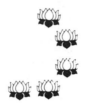

THE CHAKRA PAINTINGS reproduced on the color plate pages are original paintings done under my direction in 1970.

However, the symbolism and style are traditional, and the use of such symbol-complex images is important in all spiritual traditions.

Exoterically, such illustrations are similar to parables—they are used to describe certain concepts and principles, and then to bring them together in a *holographic* image that acts much like a multi-dimensional recording. Each element of the illustrations, i.e. the Sanskrit letters, the images of God and Goddess, the animal forms, etc. brings to the whole its own set of associated "facts" and feelings. As a composite image, these individual elements are brought together in a relationship that reveals new factors and excites new feelings, and those in turn open "psychic doors" to forgotten memories and even into the Collective Unconscious (the Astral Light of Occultism) for the memories and knowledge of the entire human (and supra-human) race.

Esoterically, such illustrations are magical. Visualized, meditated upon, energized with devotion and with wonder, they become three-dimensional holographs that can do amazing things to the psychic (and even to the neural!) circuitry of the body/soul complex. New pathways in the physical brain and in the non-physical are opened up. New psychic "organs" may be created.

This is *Spiritual Technology* only hinted at in previous texts, secrets hidden from view because of their power to transform the Human into the supra-human: the power by which men become Gods.

In Tantric sexual practice, to see your partner as divine— *to actually and deliberately worship and adore the divine in your sexual partner—* is to initiate the process of transformation.

Use the commentaries on each of the chakra paintings as "seeds" for your own meditations while looking at the illustrations. When you become familiar with them so that you can visualize them, do so and make them three-dimensional and look at those images from all sides. Let them trigger access to new information and arouse new feelings. Return to the illustrations, correct your visualizations, enrich them with the details you missed previously, and let them grow in your psyche.

MULADHARA: "ROOT BASE"
(see Chakra One color plate)

The yellow square is the element earth, bestowing solidarity and cohesiveness. This stability is further reinforced by the seven-trunked royal elephant, "Airavata," who reappears in Vishuddhi chakra with but one trunk.

Airavata's seven trunks represent the tantric potential of Muladhara to awaken the other six chakras (although the seventh chakra, Sahasrara, is really an amalgamation of the first six centers).

Thus these trunks remind us of the latent power within Muladhara that can spread through olfaction, or odor, as the quickest erotic trigger mechanism affecting the entire subtle anatomy.

Muladhara contains the Shakti energy, as Kundalini, coiled three and a half times, serpent-like, around the elliptical, phallic Shiva Lingam. In some representations the serpent, Kundalini, encapsulates the head of the Shiva Lingam—an esoteric reference to the psychic efficacy of oral congress.

In terms of human sexuality, Muladhara works synergistically with Swadhisthana, the second chakra. Muladhara is the control and arousal switch for tumescence and detumescence of erectile tissue; i.e. nasal lining, the nipples and the genitals.

Brahma, as lord of creation and procreation, generation and regeneration, sits upon the elephant's head. Lord Brahma is five-headed, each head representing an ultimate aspect of being as indicated by the prefix of the sacred syllable *Om.* His being is:

1. OM-nifarious (including all things)
2. OM-nipotent (all powerful)
3. OM-nivorous (all devouring)
4. OM-nipresent (everywhere at once)
5. OM-niscient (all knowing)

Herein is the secret meaning of the Pranava, or mantra

Om, which manifests nakedly in Ajna, the sixth chakra.

Upon Brahma's right is the feminine doorkeeper for the compressed energies of Muladhara. Her name is Dakini and she is mistress of the skin—a hint that in a state of tantric arousal the entire dermal surface becomes one extended pulsating, psychic genital.

The Bija mantra *Lam* (pronounced "lum") appears as a gold Sanskrit letter, inside the yellow yantra of earth. This is the primal palatal sound, awakening the licentious, libidinous, lascivious force of Muladhara as the phallic tongue reverberates within the vaginal oral cavity.

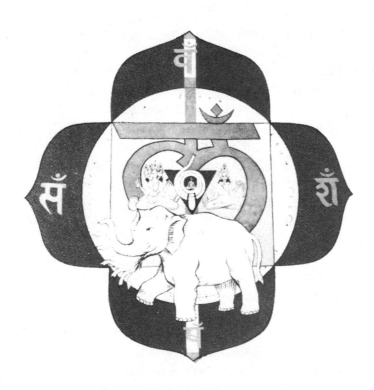

SWADHISTHANA: "ONE'S OWN PLACE"
(see Chakra Two color plate)

The second center controls the ocean of fluids within the human aquarium. This includes the saline blood, lymph, bile, urine, perspiration, saliva, semen, menstrual blood, breast milk, vaginal secretions (during sexual arousal), and lubricant secretions from the duct glands of male and female genitals.

When erotically stimulated, alchemical dew is exudated from capillaries lining the vaginal wall, in the same way that cerebral spinal fluid is constantly secreted from capillaries lining the hollow brain ventricles. "As above so below."

The fire-breathing crocodile is a mythical beast called "Makara." He is the vehicle of Varuna—lord of cosmic waters, and also the mount of the goddess Ganga. the Makara appears on the banner of Kama—the Indian Cupid. Ritual consumption of crocodile genitals, as an aphrodisiac, is still practiced in many parts of the world.

The lunar phase, locked in with the monthly menstrual cycle (month comes from Latin *menses*) is seen as a half moon supporting the Sanskrit letter for the sound *Vam* (pronounced "wum"), mantra of water vibration.

Housed in the Sanskrit cypher nestle the God and Goddess, separated by the golden pillar of the middle way, called *Shushumna,* or the "royal path."

Vishnu is upon the reader's left. He is the preserver of life and, in a physiological context, maintains the homeostasis of body fluids; e.g. blood.

Rakini, the Shakti, is the queen of blood and liquids. Concerning the two-headed Rakini, the Shatchakra Nirupana states, "and from one of her nostrils flows a streak of blood (perhaps a reference to the vicarious menstruation of the pubescent girl). She is fond of white rice (a hygroscopic or fluid-retaining substance) and grants the wished for boon" (the power of orgasmic sex magic).

MANIPURA: "JEWEL CITY"
(see Chakra Three color plate)

The third chakra, Manipura, has fire—psychic and physical—as the element of jurisdiction. At the gross level this includes all metabolic processes of the body, and in particular, activity of the liver and pancreas.

At a more subtle level, Manipura channels sensations from the activated "abdominal brain" or solar plexus. It is at the sun nexus that we experience the molten lava of passion, buried under the mountain of the diaphragm, and volcanically spewing forth as lust, power and drive.

The animal ("Great Beast") is the ram or Mesha, battering down all obstacles with the holy flames of enthusiasm. Mesha is sometimes seen as the "horned goat of Mendes," and "to ride the goat" is to control the powerful forces inherent in this center.

The god on the right is Rudra (Lord of the tempest), a prototype of Shiva (the transformer). Rudra is known also as "the Lord of tears," for tears flow both with the agony and the ecstasy of sexual passion. Such lacrimal floods subdue overactivity of Manipura, restoring etheric and physical equipoise.

The Devi is Lakini: ruler of all flesh, three-headed, and dweller within the live-r, controller of the pancreas, Greek *pan* (all) and *creas* (flesh).

The pink Sanskrit letter in front of the red triangle is *Ram* (pronounced "rum"), a power resonance related to the magic fire of "Amon-Ra," the occult key to closing invocations with "Amen."

The red triangle, apex down, is a female Shakti symbol of the burning yoni, the wand's chalice: the physical and spiritual portal to life after life.

ANAHATA: "UNSTRUCK SOUND"
(see Chakra Four color plate)

The fourth astral vortex is related to the heart, perpetual motion, and that section of the *Atom-sphere (Atmosphere)* we breathe.

At Anahata, the second great Yoga (union) takes place in the journey from womb to tomb. The newborn's first inhalation sets the heart and lung rhythm into synchronicity through activation of the cardio-pulmonary plexus. Ever after the normal respiratory cycle of inhalation and exhalation, in proportion to the number of heartbeats, will be a constant ratio of one to four. Four heartbeats for every respiration cycle is the magic essence of those occult breathing methods in which the breath is retained for four times as long as the inhalation.

The antelope is associated with Anahata as typifying alertness and sensitivity, exactly as the heartbeat and respiration change with every signal from the environment.

Indra, Indo-Aryan chief of the gods, tantrically indentified with the power of the Lingam as phallus, is shown on the left. He is here depicted blue-skinned, but often represented as covered with Yonis as punishment for a sexual indiscretion. This latter form is a tantric implication about the sensory outlet for Anahata: the exquisitely sensitive tactile receptors of the genitals and nipples.

This sensory expression of tactile receptors links Anahata with Muladhara—in fact we could say Anahata is the "Muladhara" of the first of the chakras above the diaphragm. Consider how many women are capable of having a climax from nipple stimulation only! It is Nature's closed loop feedback system to reinforce breast feeding.

The relationship between Anahata and Muladhara is strengthened by Anahata's traditional command of the procreative function.

The four-headed female deity is Kakini; she has sovereignty over body fats including cholesterol and ketones.

The blue interlocked triangles, the shatkona (literally "six angled" figure) subsumes all unions including mind and body, conscious and unconscious, male and female (female superior position demonstrated by the female triangle, apex down). This latter concept is emphasized by the gold Sanskrit letter *Yam* (pronounced "yum") as in Tibetan *yab-yum* translated as "Father-Mother face."

The heart, as the physical center of Anahata, is the temple upon the mountain of the diaphragm, and here the chela transmutes the passion of Manipura to the compassion of Anahata. Sexual lust is distilled into love, and sexual pair bonding results.

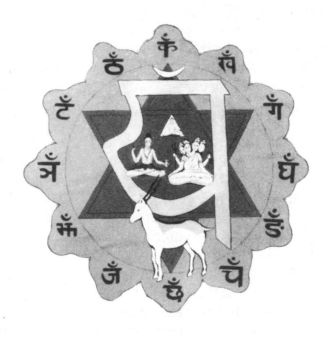

THE ASANAS
OF LOVE

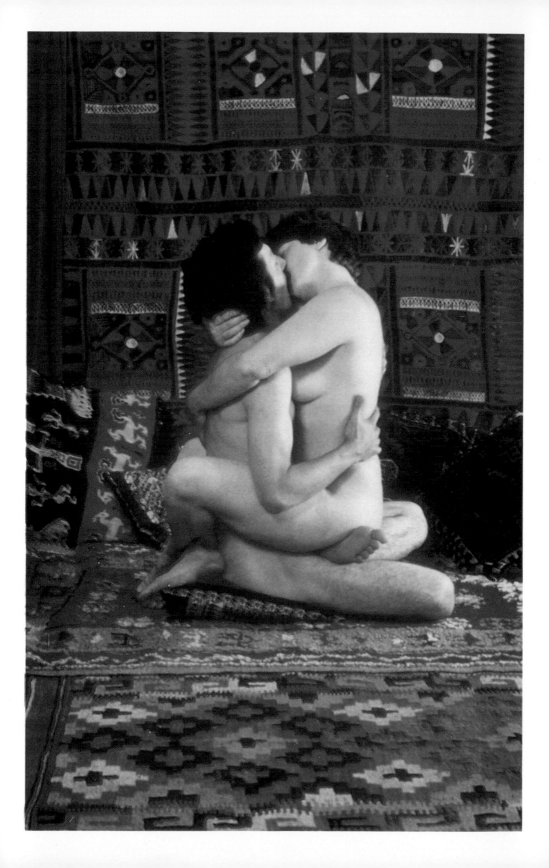

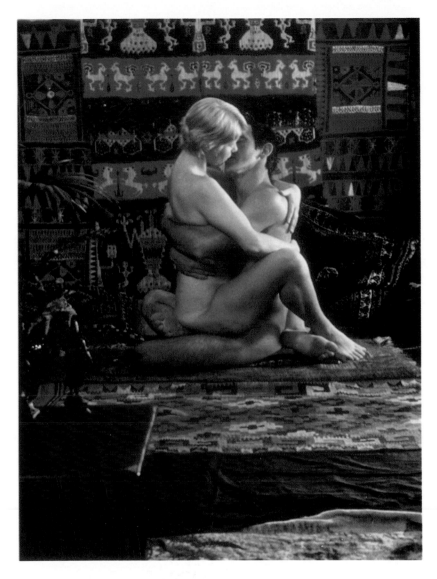

YAB YUM (Father-Mother)

The male sits locked in lotus posture with the female sitting atop him, her legs clinging around his hips. The penis is deeply and securely inserted in the vagina, while the 'Father Face' and 'Mother Face' are locked together with tongues touching firmly and arms strongly hugging each close to the other. This is an ideal posture for 'pre-birth rocking' until the moment of orgasm. The man may find additional support from a pillow placed under his buttocks.

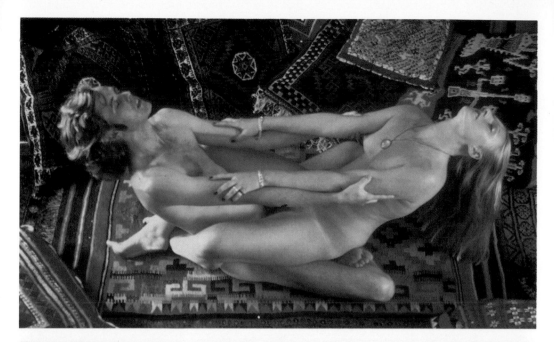

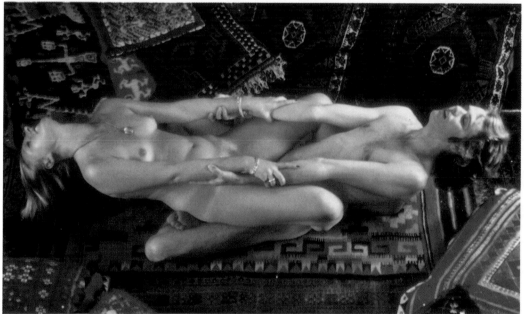

MULA BANDHA (Root or Basal Lock)

The man is in full lotus or the much simpler *sukhasana* (crossed leg) posture with the woman astride, legs firmly entwined around and behind his hips, her heels wedged between the floor and the sacral area of his spine when he leans back supine. Shakta and Shakti firmly clasp wrists and each leans back giving support to the other until both are supine or face up. Psychic fire is built to ejaculation by focusing on the slow friction of the Lingam in the Yoni as the partners gently pull each other into an upright position and lower themselves again repeatedly until climax.

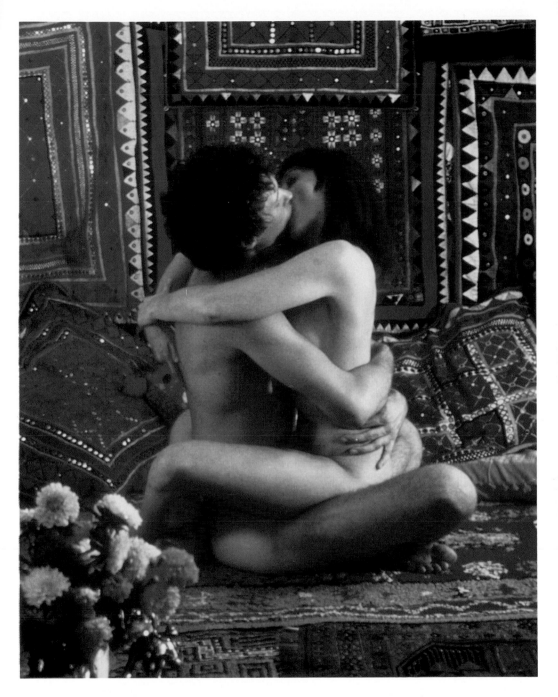

SUKHAPADMA ASANA (Easy Lotus Posture)
Lord Shiva's legs are comfortably crossed in the half lotus or just crossed 'tailor fashion', with Shakti mounted on him, her legs wrapped firmly around his waist. All psychic circuits are closed—so that they interlock tongue to tongue, breast to breast, navel to navel, with Lingam keyed into the lock of Yoni.

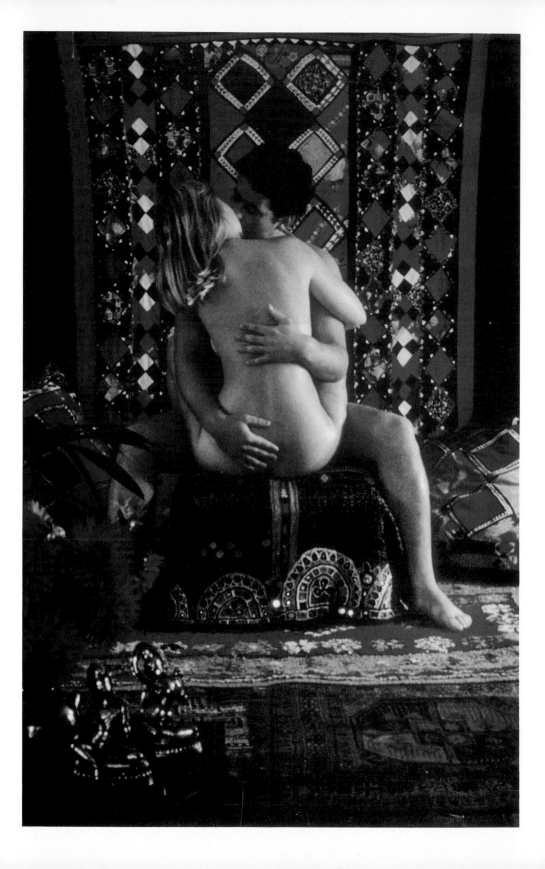

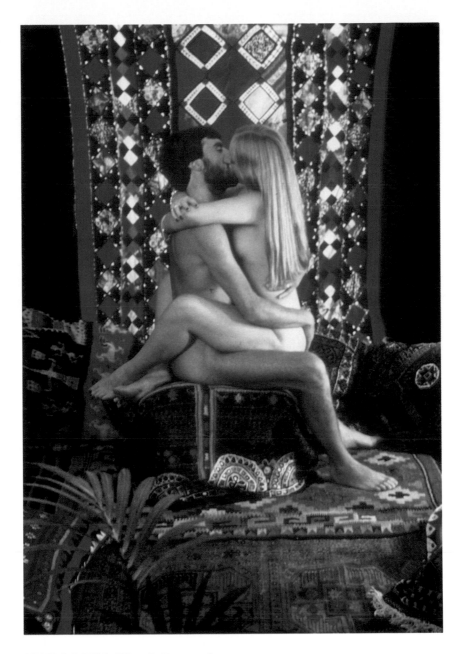

YONI ASANA (Womb Posture)
The man sits in a chair or upon a couch with his legs bent at the knees, resting the soles of his feet on the floor. The woman is seated in his lap, yoked to him sexually and with her arms entwined around his neck. Her steadiness of position is assisted by his embrace.

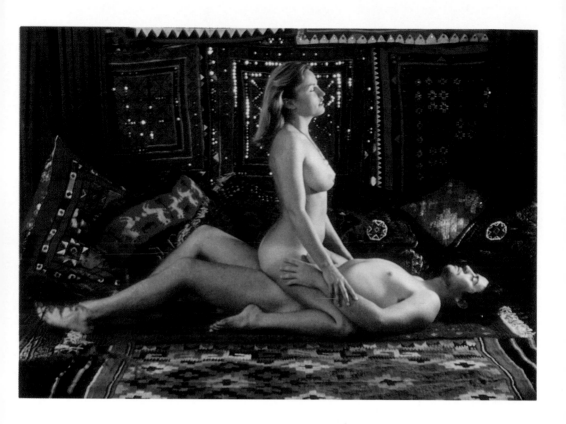

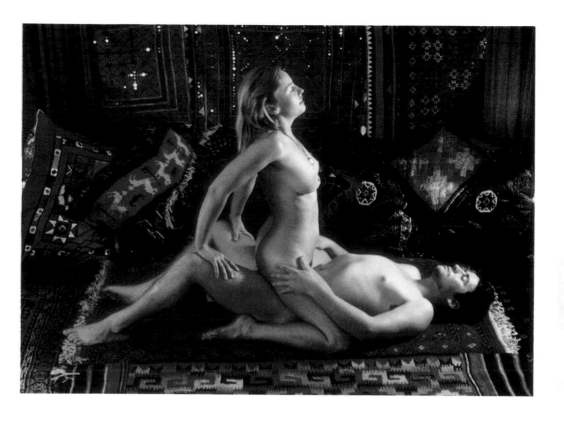

KALI ASANA (Kali's Pose)
also **VIPARITAKARANI (Reverse Action)**

The man lies down face up with the woman surmounting and riding him. She clasps his Lingam in her Yoni, using the powerful vaginal muscles to massage and milk him. Her clitoris is freely exposed to digital stimulation by him, which almost guarantees simultaneous orgasms. *Kali asana* is noted for producing particularly strong vaginal sensations because of the stretch applied to the front wall of the vagina by the penis, which is forcibly pulled back from a normal forty-five degree angle.

THE
CHAKRAS

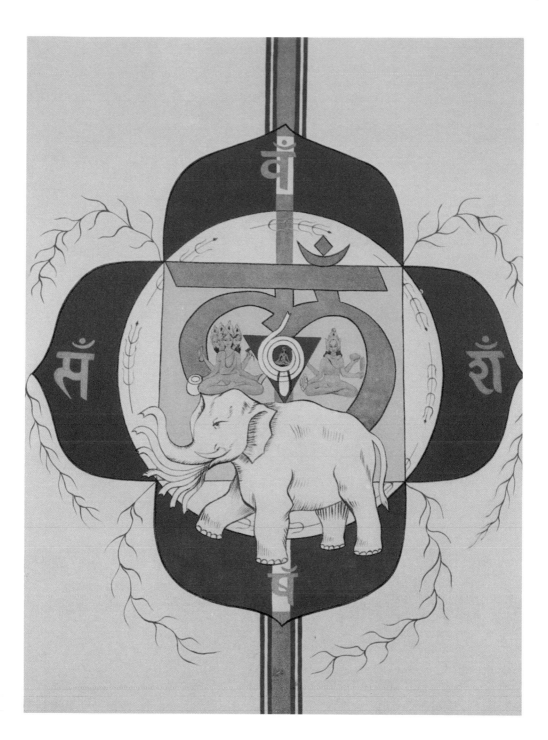

MULADHARA CHAKRA

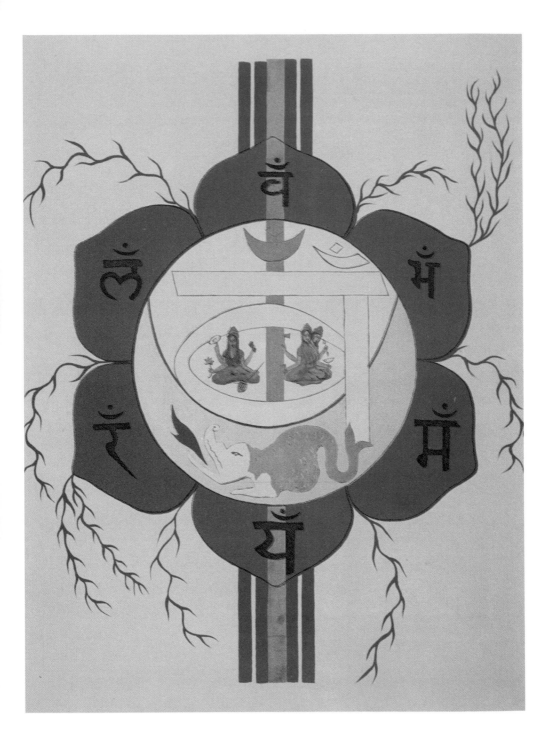

SWADHISTHANA CHAKRA

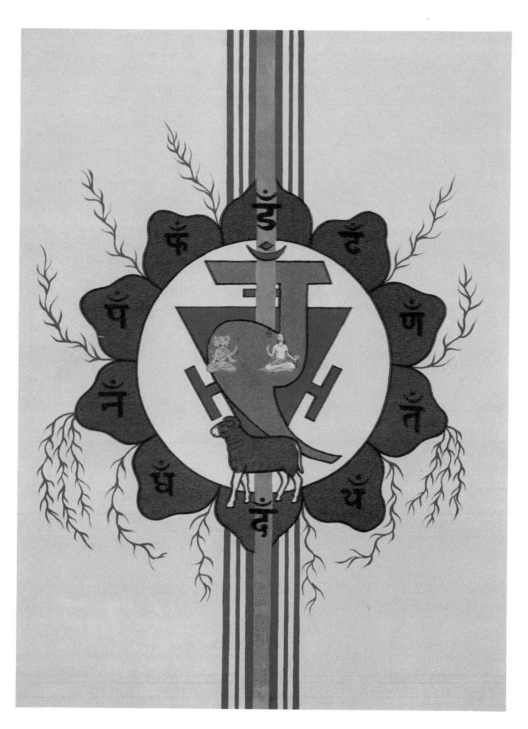

MANIPURA CHAKRA

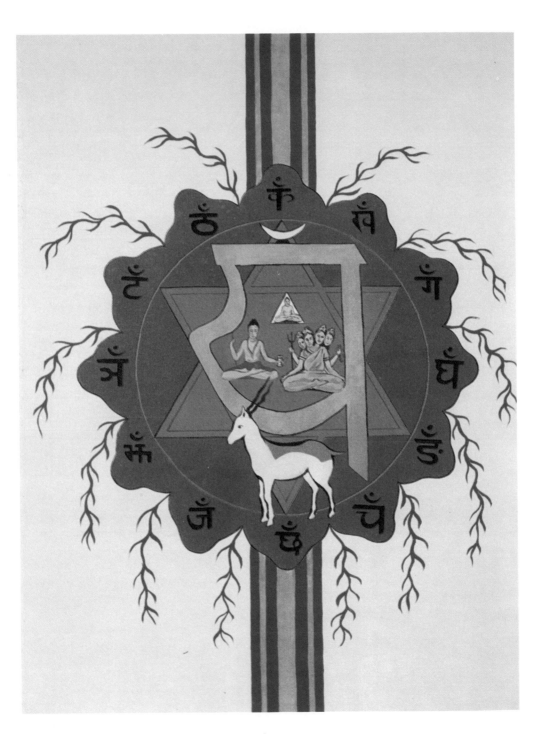

ANAHATA CHAKRA

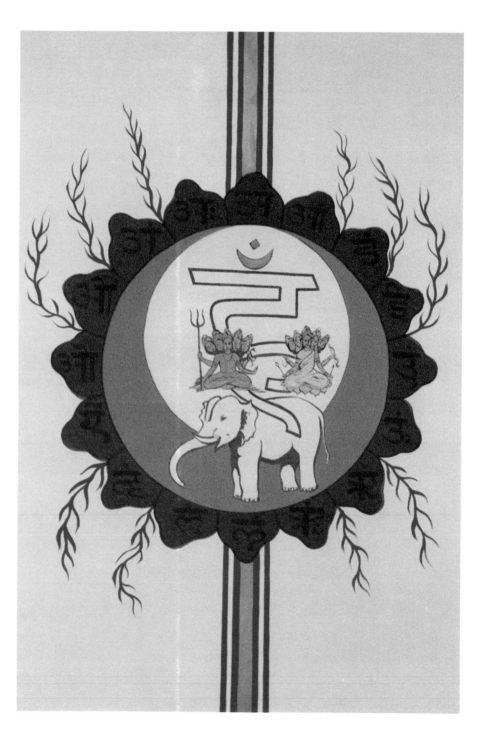

VISHUDDHI CHAKRA

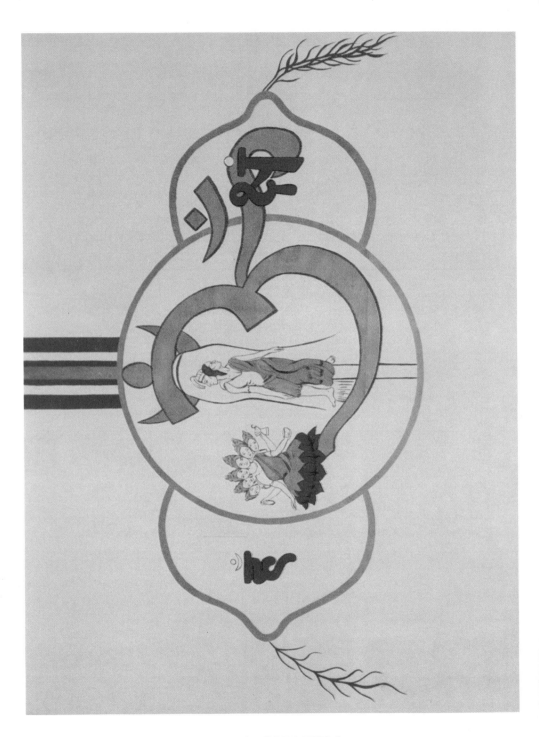

AJNA CHAKRA

VISHUDDHI: "WITH PURITY"
(see Chakra Five color plate)

Vishuddhi demarcates the mundane from the arcane. Astral energy progressing through this chakra undergoes transubstantiation, becoming Soma or Amrita, respectively, the psychedelic drink of the priests and the elixir of immortality for the Gods. The initiate at Vishuddhi converts the compassion of Anahata into *empathy*—the Buddha-like resonance with all sentient beings.

Located at the base of the throat, this chakra manifests in the physical body as the thyroid and parathyroid glands, the pharyngeal plexus, speech and hearing (paired as "deaf and dumb").

Speech and hearing coalesce, with Tantric climax, producing involuntary mantric utterances, "speaking in tongues," and psychic deafness. Male and female neophytes become adepts, and experience a shift from mundane *no-where* to *now-here!*

The associated element is ether (Akasha). Ether includes the entire energy spectrum from outer space cosmic rays, through to the electro-magnetic gamut. Akasha is shown as the Chandra Poornima or full moon set against an oval blue background. Frequently the black egg of infinite space is used as a symbol of Akasha.

Sadashiva (Lord of transformation), five-headed, is above the "pure" albino royal elephant. Sadashiva holds a trident (Trishula) as a sign of the tantric nuclear triad. The triad is spermatazoa, ovum and their mutual intercourse, producing the magical child of Thoth. Such a conjunction is the first great Yoga, predating individual existence.

The Shakti is Shakini, her five heads representing the five lower senses, the basis of mundane existence for the uninitiated.

"She lives in bone and feasts upon milk"
—*Shat Chakra Nirupana*

Although this suggests an intuitive grasp of calcium as the foundation of the skeletal matrix, and the parathyroids' function in calcium metabolism, for the occultist milk means tantric potions of semen, soma, and lacteal secretions.

Shiva and Shakini have behind them the white Sanskrit letter for the seed sound *Ham* (pronounced "Hum"). Devotees intoning this vibration, while locked together in maithuna, transcend the eternal cycle of birth and rebirth. Esoterically, rebirth is the incessant round of thought after thought giving birth to yet another thought. The mantra *Hum* freezes the wheel of Samsara in the void of Akasha, thus bringing into fruition Patanjali's injunction:

> *Yoga is the cessation of*
> *the fluctuations of the mind-stuff.*

AJNA: "COMMAND CENTER"
(see Chakra Six color plate)

Ajna is the last of the Shat (six) chakras. Among Ajna's many epithets is *Divya Chaksu*—literally, divine eye.

Ajna is the alpha and omega, the polar opposite of Muladhara, having as its element mind or *Manas.*

All of the prior sensory avenues are dependent upon Manas, and the real genitals reside within the relaxed, receptive consciousness open to messages from the erogenous zones. Love must fill the hermetic crucible of the skull for transubstantiation to occur.

The two petals on either side of the circle are as wings to a world globe. They symbolize imagination, which takes flight across the universe to penetrate other dimensions.

The right petal (reader's left) frames the red letter *Ha* (the sun) while the left petal holds *K'sha,* a conjunct consonant, which is the occult (eclipsing) sign of *Tha,* the moon. Thus *HaTha* yoga is the celestial marriage of sun and moon, mind and body, Adam and Eve, leading to the opening of the third *eye* and the evolved "sixth sense." "Mind over matter" becomes a manifest actuality.

The gold Mukta Bija (freedom seed sound) *Om* occupies the central Manas circle. Chanting *Om* elicits wandering in stellar space with subjective re-instatement of Lord Brahma's attributes. That which is below (Muladhara) consubstantiates with that which is above (Ajna). "As above so below."

Paramshiva (highest aspect of transformation) is contained within the phallic thumb. The deity is androgynous, as the penultimate archetype of bisexual cosmic consciousness. Paramshiva co-exists as both hermaphrodite (Mercury and Venus in conjunction) and virgin (from the Greek, giving such English words as *virile* and *gynaecology*). The tantric, having achieved wholeness (holiness) in Ajna, surrenders awareness of gender differentiation (e.g., is again a "virgin") and engages in the back-to-back witch dance throughout eternal time and across infinite space.

To Paramshiva's left is Hakini, also known as Siddhakali, "the accomplished mother of death." She has six heads corresponding to the five lower senses and the sixth sense of enlightened humanity.

This sixth sense is intuition (inner tutor), the consequence of a yoga between the right and left hemispheres of the brain. The feminine, receptive, right hemisphere processes information and flashes the conclusion across to the masculine, logical left hemisphere, producing an altered state of consciousness experienced as a sudden gestalt or "Eureka!" grasp of reality.

The universal phallic thumb, from which Paramshiva emerges, is called "Kama kala," the love digit. The English word "thumb" comes from the same Indo-Aryan Germanic root that gives us "tumescence," the engorgement of genital tissue accompanying piercing of "being" with the arrows released from the bow of Eros. The love digit indicates the relationship between tantric control of sexual experience and the opening of the Ajna chakra. Our colloquialism "under the thumb" suggests the secret.

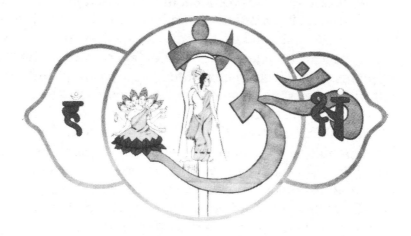

Sexual Terminology: Semantics of the Inner Life

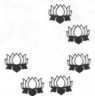

THE SYSTEM OF Tantra I teach emphasizes study of psycholinguistics (the influence of language on individual behavior), etymology (word origins) and semantics (levels of meaning). The major aspects of occultism, Eastern and Western, may be unraveled through research into Sanskrit, Hebrew, Greek and Latin. In dealing with language as a key for unlocking esoteric knowledge, I have developed a number of auxiliary principles, including the following:

ONOMATOPOEIA

The more suggestive in sound of the action or object a word represents, the more potent the word is. Some languages exhibit this quality more frequently than others. For instance, the English word "peace," denoting calmness and tranquillity, is phonetically or vibrationally quite inept compared with the Sanskrit equivalent, "shanti." The English "p" is a forceful

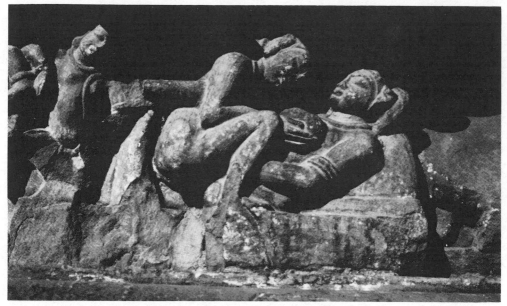

Lakshmana Temple, Khajuraho.

and sudden plosive sound (note our word "explosive"), which in "peace" encourages, we could conjecture, the typically Western aggressive attitude, "We will have peace if we have to fight for it." Compare the soft, sibilant Sanskrit "shanti," possessing a sound unconsciously utilized in the English use of "shush" or "sssh," to obtain quiet and silence.

CURRENT MEANING VERSUS ORIGINAL ROOT MEANING

English is a dynamic, ever-changing language, in which the original meanings of most words have long been forgotten and the same words are now used with different connotations. "Cunning" has a derogatory implication suggestive of slyness or trickery, yet in the Middle English of the thirteenth to fifteenth century, it meant simply one who was knowing.

"Conjuration," which we now associate with an incantation, spell or charm, is of Latin origin and in Shakespeare's time meant the act of swearing on an oath or making a solemn appeal, which in a sense could be considered a binding obligation or "spell."

A "wit" (from the Sanskrit root *vid*, "to see," intact in English as "video") was not a humorist six hundred years ago but rather "a wise man." This context of the word is still evident in such popular expressions as "sharpening your wits" and "keeping your wits about you."

Frozen languages such as Sanskrit, used for religious scriptures rather than for everyday vernacular, are more dependable linguistically as they can preserve precise meanings across the centuries.

ANAGRAMS

This is the magical doctrine of the Cabala, called Temurah, in which phrases or words formed from the letters of another word or motto are related and unveil new levels of insight.

"Veda" is a Sanskrit term signifying "knowing," "understanding," and "perceiving." The Vedas are classical texts of Hinduism representing, as the title indicates, embodied wisdom. "Veda," by the process of Temurah, transposes into "Deva," "shining one," i.e., a god. "Deva" is the Sanskrit source of our English "Deity" and "Divine." The great Hermetic axiom, "As above, so below," is clearly exemplified, as he who possesses wisdom (veda) becomes a god (Deva). God is man!

As a more sophisticated example, let us take the letters in the word "love," out of which we can form "vole," a variant of the more common French *voler*, to fly ("in seventh heaven") and related to our English "volatile." "Vole" is also to risk everything in a game of chance, to "risk all for love"; "it is better to have loved and lost than never to have loved at all," etc. Finally, *vole* is a Scandinavian word assimilated into English meaning a "field mouse," and if you wonder what that has to do with "love," allow your mind to roam over the implications of a mouse's propensity for secreting itself in hidden recesses, cavities and holes. This is the reason Lord Ganesha, the elephant-headed God of Wisdom in Hindu mythology, has as his helper a rat. Puzzled? Ganesha's trunk is a phallic symbol—which says a great deal about where the Hindus feel wisdom resides.

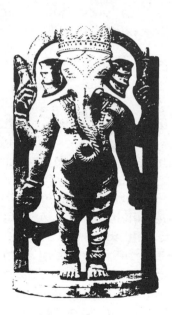

ASSONANCE AND CLANG ASSOCIATIONS

Assonance is the association of words because of a similarity in vowel sounds, e.g., devil and revel, altar and alter. Closely related are clang associations in which words sounding alike are associationally linked, e.g., bang and twang, Tantra and Mantra. Both assonance and clang associations are prominent features of some psychotic thought processes. However, they can be useful for connecting terms meaningfully that have no direct linguistic relationship to each other.

Consider the Sanskrit "Shakti," which refers to power and energy, feminine in quality, manifested in nature or the macrocosm and latent in man, the microcosm, coiled at the sacral (Latin for "sacred") base of the spine. When the Shakti or Kundalini is aroused, tradition states that an epileptiform trembling of the body commences, which is reminiscent of the tonic and clonic vibrations of the thigh marking a full orgasm. The only word in English similar to "Shakti" is "shake." To understand the full implications of Shakti, use the word "shake" to go on an ideational flight which rapidly encompasses the Shakers, an offshoot of the English 17th century Quakers and later another related American sect, the Holy Rollers, all groups giving evidence that the ecstatic state of Shakti's uniting with Lord Shiva is a state of autonomic nervous system excitability discharging as "the shakes."

Free association, magical thinking (believing that thoughts and wishes have power—a belief characteristic of thought processes in children up to about age six), flights of ideas, and neologisms (formation of new words to express subjective states) are also valuable adjuncts of the occultist when exploring linguistics. This is understandable when we realize that the magician, the artist and the psychotic all share a common psychological ground called autism. As defined by Bleuler, one of Freud's colleagues, autism is a detachment from reality with relative and absolute predominance of the inner life. In autism the content of thought is determined more by fantasies and wishes than by the demands and realities of everyday thinking. Cultivation of autism permits plumbing the depths of creativity in the mind.

AMRITA: in Hindu mythology, a juice or nectar which is the elixir of life. The Sanskrit prefix *a* denotes "not," "no," "against," while the root *mrta* means "dead." *Mrta* is cognate with Latin *morte,* as found in the English "mortal," "postmortem" and "moribund." Amrita is the drink of immortality.

Tantric doctrine conceives that Amrita is manufactured in the alchemical laboratory of the body through the fires of sustained sexual excitement.

In Western physiology it is acknowledged that sexual sensations of sufficient intensity may stimulate the pituitary-pineal-hypothalamic complex, throwing rare hormones into the bloodstream. A typical example occurs in women when nipple stimulation triggers the pituitary gland, which in turn releases a substance producing uterine contractions. Breast feeding post-natally helps shrink the uterus. Indeed, some women can have an orgasm by manipulation of the breast alone.

Doctors Masters and Johnson have demonstrated that the vaginal walls secrete a dew under sexual stimulus. David Reuben *(Everything You Wanted to Know About Sex . . .)* mentions lowered incidence of arthritis and rheumatism among those enjoying frequent orgasms, and Dr. E. Scheimann *(Sex and the Overweight Woman)* points out that men with sexual frustrations are much more apt to have heart attacks.

Tantra has recognized for thousands of years that sexual activity is a key to rejuvenation, and Amrita consists of a series of biochemical substances produced by the endocrine glands and mucous membranes of the body in response to sustained erotic ritual.

CLIMAX: used as a term for the desirable culmination of sexual stimulation, "climax" comes from the Greek *klimax,* meaning a "ladder or staircase to heaven," indicating the inner significance of sexuality as a spiritual path. This is unconsciously implicit in the joke that a "run" in nylon stockings or pantyhose is "a ladder to heaven."

CLITORIS: from Greek through Latin, as in *clavis,* a "key." The term refers to that part of the female vulva which unlocks a women's nervous system in the same way that a key unlocks a door.

CONSUMMATE: used in the contemporary sense of completing a marriage through intercourse. The original Latin root is replete with the significance of the esoteric object of intercourse, for to consummate is to bring to completion (Yoga), or perfection, to make perfect (Siddhi), to raise to the highest, topmost, utmost, and the "crown of" (the object of Tantric intercourse is to open Sahasrara, the "crown" chakra).

CREATE: From the Sanskrit root *kr* meaning "to make," through Latin, as in *creare,* implying production, growing, to bring into existence. The close relationship between sexual fecundity and mental originality is demonstrated by our use of the word "create" to denote both the creation of life and artistic creativity.

The birth of ideas is an analog to physical birth. We use words like "conceiving" and "conception" interchangeably for either physical pregnancy or mental agility. We also speak of a "fertile woman" and a "fertile imagination."

Occult psychology views the mind as divided into the masculine, active consciousness and the feminine, passive unconscious. The art of mental creation is an alchemical process of impregnating the unconscious mind with a seed or germinal idea grasped by consciousness but ejaculated into the deeper unconscious realms for incubation. Gestation continues in the unconscious womb until the sudden birth of the idea as a "flash" or "inspiration" as it emerges fully formed into consciousness.

DELIRIUM: composed of Latin *lira,* a "furrow," and *de,* the Latin preposition "out of" or "from." Delirium is "going out of the furrow," "off the track," "deviating from, leaving the straight line."

In Yoga and Western magic this is a desirable state of transcendent consciousness in which the practitioner is out of the "rut" of so-called normality with its attendant limitations. After all, the difference between a rut and a grave is a mere matter of degree!

ECSTASY: "I stand outside" (myself) from the Greek prefix *ex* (out) and *stasis* (a standing). "Ecstasy" refers to a state of supraconsciousness outside the little "self" or petty "ego," in short, "a trip" away from the mundane framework of daily mental existence.

EROS: the Greek God of Love. The word comes from an earlier Sanskrit root *Aris,* meaning to be filled with desire or zeal. In English, the derivatives from the Greek

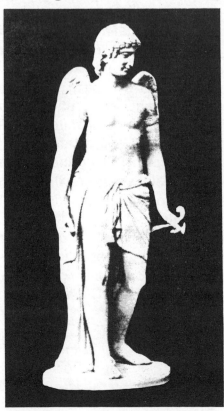

include "erotic" (amatory desire), "erogenous" (sensitive zones of the body arousing sexual desire), "eroticism" (sexual orientation) and "erotomania" (pathological awareness of sexual passion).

By Temurah we form the anagram "rose" from "eros." The rose was sacred to Aphrodite (Greek Goddess of Love; hence "aphrodisiac" for a sexual stimulant), for she pricked her feet upon rose thorns searching for her slain lover, Ares, the God of War. The relationship between Aphrodite (the Roman Venus) and Ares (the Roman Mars) is an allegory of the ambivalence love and hate build into all intimate liaisons. Eros gave a rose to Harpocrates, God of Silence, to keep him from revealing the indiscretions of Venus, which is a warning to practitioners of sex magic and Tantra about the necessity for silence as a guarantee of ritual potency. The ancient Romans suspended a rose from the ceiling at dinner parties with the understanding that conversation under the rose was confidential, or as the lawyer says, "sub rosa."

Lastly, "eros" becomes "sore," the modern English deriving from the Anglo-Saxon *sar,* meaning "painful," "wounded," the etymology being a reminder that nothing is obtained or attained without payment. Illumination through passion, on the path to compassion, exacts its own price.

MAD: in describing this word, the Oxford dictionary uses as synonyms "rabid," "wildly foolish," "reckless," "keen," and "infatuated." Sanskrit "mad" is either the source or a cognate entwining through Old High German into Anglo-Saxon and thence into modern English. The Sanskrit is closest to the sense of "mad" in "divine madness," for it means "intoxicated with joy," "excitement," "inspiration," "a soma (psychedelic drug) draught," "exhilarated," while the variant "madud" means to be "out of one's senses with excitement," and "to be frantic."

The conceptual triad of "delirium," "ecstasy" and

"madness" refers to desirable religious experiences in which consciousness is heightened. Going "mad" may bring enlightenment, something modern psychiatry is being forced to recognize through the efforts of R. D. Laing and his school of "anti-psychiatry." Tantra, Yoga, Buddhism and Western ceremonial magic systematically bring about insanity to evolve more sanity or wholeness.

"Mad" backwards is "dam." Ecstasy is the bursting of the dam or locks which protect the ego and consciousness from being overwhelmed by the unconscious torrents within us all. The Tantrist deliberately removes the "dam" between consciousness and the unconscious when he has achieved sufficient discipline to contain the madness. The psychotic, through mishap of genes and environment, has the dam shattered prematurely and consequently drowns in the turbulence of his own mad mind. "Adm," the father of mankind, whose name is another anagram of mad, has seeded within us all "divine madness." Tantra breaches the dam with sexual ecstasy, flooding planes of consciousness normally arid.

ORGASM: found in English through French and Latin from two closely related Greek roots. *Orgio,* a sacred rite, sacrifice (of semen?), ceremony in the early Greco-Roman mysteries celebrating the feast of Dionysus or Bacchus; hence our expression "an orgy." *Orgasio,* the second related root, means to swell, with ardent desire or passion (expansion of an auric field similar to the way a balloon is overinflated), to burst. The roots suggest an experience of such intense excitement that the ego is momentarily fragmented, producing a nameless-formless inner state.

PHALLUS: a Greek term originating with the earlier Sanskrit *phal,* which has the semantically pregnant meaning "to burst," "to split." A variation is the Sanskrit *phalanti,* "to bear fruit." Both Greek and Sanskrit derivatives may be related to the English "pole," which derives from the Phoenician word meaning "he breaks through" or "passes into." Maypole dancing is a vestigial trace of an ancient fertility rite in which the phallic pole penetrates the vaginal Earth.

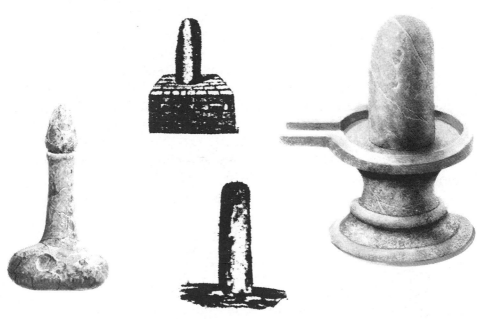

A graphic portrayal of the penis as an object of veneration is found in both Greek Dionysian and Hindu Shiva cults. The phallus is the ultimate symbol of creative power in the manifest universe. The spellbinding aspect of the penis as a magical wand or scepter is demonstrated by the word "fascinate," which comes from a Latin base simultaneously referring to the male organ and witchcraft.

Freud alerted the European mind to the sexual duality of all objects in terms of shape. Everything that is elongated, pointed and projecting is masculine and phallic. Rounded, enclosing, curving forms are feminine symbols unconsciously mimicking the womb and breasts.

Freud's American disciple, the analyst A. A. Brill,

observed awareness of this symbology deeply embedded in the racial unconscious of little boys preparing for adult roles by endlessly jamming pencils into keyholes. By contrast, little girls, in unconscious anticipation of being future recipients of the penis, seldom manifest an urge to pierce objects or ram apertures with rods.

While on the subject of pencils and penises, it is a pity those men needlessly anxious about the size of their genitals are not aware that any woman can obtain complete orgasmic satisfaction masturbating with her little finger or any object the diameter of a pencil, including a pencil.

SACRUM: the triangular "sacred bone" (Latin *sacrare*) at the base of the spine which forms the posterior portion of the pelvis. The vertebral column known as the "Staff of God" (Brahma-dandu) in Tantra rests upon the sacrum. The sacrum, in Yoga literature, is called the Kanda (meaning "root") or Trikona (tri-angle). It consists of five fused vertebrae in the adult. The "sacred" nerves running off the spinal cord like branches from a tree (the brain and spinal cord represent the tree of knowledge mentioned in Genesis) are the major nerve fibers awakening the uterus, cervix, vagina, prostate gland and penis into activity.

The ancients knew of the connection between sexual arousal and the nerves emerging from the sacrum, and for them, copulation was sacred and consecrated rather than profane.

SEX: from the Latin *sexus*, literally meaning "division," possibly from *sec-are*, meaning "to cut." Existence of the "sexes" implies a prior cutting or separation which is only re-paired by sexual communion (communication). This act of copulation (coupling) is the essential yoking bringing about a state of "Yoga."

The English *sexeneal* (the Latin *sexenium*), a period

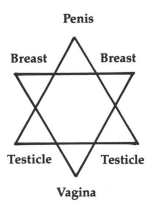

of six years, is an equivalent or cognate of the Greek prefix *hex,* meaning "six." A hexagram is the six-pointed star, the Judaic Star of David and the Hindu Vishnu Yantra. Esoterically, the hexagram is a geometrical diagram of intercourse depicting the union of the male triangle (mind or Adam) with the female triangle (body or Eve). In Tantra, the six points of the star are the major genital erogenic zones of male and female. The hexagram, if we may be permitted a neologism, is really a "sexagram."

SEX MAGIC: Sex magic operates upon the premise that whatever is held in the imagination at the moment of orgasm will come to pass. Expressing this concept in another way: the mind is like a computer which will solve any problem presented, provided that the problem is "fed" at the optimum moment when the machine is switched on and warmed up, i.e., when easy access to the unconscious is possible. Orgasm occurs at such a moment when the conscious mind is quelled, freeing the unconscious.

The difference between sex magic and other systems stilling the conscious mind (meditation, ceremonial magic, and witchcraft) may be likened to the difference between the jet speed and efficiency of piloting the "whispering death" F-111 fighter, and flying a helicopter. Sex magic is more potent than other systems, but some aspects require great skill. In very advanced techniques, when something goes wrong it's like being "hit" at 20,000 feet in an F-111—you have to bale out fast, and it may cost you your life! All techniques discussed in Chapter Four are safe, contingent upon one's ability to handle the emotional and nervous energies aroused in as nonneurotic a way as possible.

TANTRA: *Tan* is a Sanskrit root meaning "thread" or "web" while *tra* signifies a "tool." One literal translation of Tantra is "thread tool"; the intricate threads composing the web of fibers in the autonomic nervous system are fired by the aroused Shakti energy coursing through them.

A more obvious and semantically fruitful translation of Tantra is "touch." Etymologically, the prefix *tan* has come into English with just that meaning. Consider the following words: "tangent," a straight line (Shiva Lingam?) touching a curved surface (Yoni?); "tango" (derived from the Latin word for "touch"), the most sensual, intimate dance; "tangible," that which we know by touch, that which is material in nature and palpable, not visionary or illusive; "tangle," an intertwined embrace; "tantalize," to excite, torture, tempt; "tantrum," a nervous outburst.

As a method for attaining supraconsciousness, Tantra utilizes the primary sensory avenue of touch, concentrating upon tactile excitation to paralyze the brain with exquisite sensation from the hypersensitive receptors embedded in the genitalia. Tantra opens the sensory gates in order to ultimately transcend both body and mind.

TESTICLE: a witness to virility, from the Latin *testis*. the words "testify," "testimony" and "testament" all spring from the same base. The ancient Hebrews swore an oath by placing their hands upon their testicles; references to this custom may be found in Genesis 24:1-9 and 48:29. The Hindus followed the same practice, swearing veracity while touching the testicles of Nanda, the temple bull sacred to Lord Shiva.

The alchemy of sex magic and Tantra begins with the elixir prepared in the personal "test tube" of the male participant.

VAGINA: Latin for "sheath," in the sense of a scabbard for a weapon. Unconscious recognition of the vagina as a "sheath" is evidenced in our language by the frequency with which the euphemisms of "weapon" and "sword" are employed for penis. From this, the Hindu

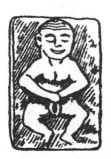

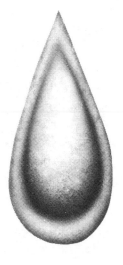

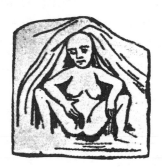

Tantric viewpoint follows that just as a sheath without a sword is valueless, so a Shakti (female) without a Shaktra (male) is worthless.

In alchemical symbology, the mortar and pestle are actually the vagina and the penis macerating the medicines of tongue, breasts and genitals.

VENERATE: allied to the Sanskrit *van,* to love or honor, but directly taken from the Latin *vener,* to revere and love. Related words from the same Latin stem are "venerable," "venereal" and "Venus" (the Roman Goddess of Love). To venerate is to recognize the sexual parts as truly worthy objects of our adoration and awe.

YONI: in Yoga and Tantra, Yoni has two meanings. It refers to the perineum of Western anatomy, the floor of the pelvis situated between the anus and the vagina or the anus and the testicles. The "Yoni Nadi" is exactly midway between these two points.
It also refers to the female vulva or external genitalia likened to a lotus bud, soft and sweet smellling. Hindu Tantric sculpture is unique among the ancient civilizations as always clearly depicting the soft curves and slit of the vulva on female nudes. I have several photographs of Tantric sculptures from the eleventh-century Hyderbad depicting a naked Goddess arched backwards, knees apart, displaying her Yoni for Puja, worshipful veneration.

Eros
and
Thanatos

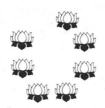

SIGMUND FREUD WAS acutely aware of the twin
drives within the human being. He drew upon a tradition as old as mankind when he termed these forces
Eros and Thanatos: Eros, the urge to love and achieve
vicarious immortality through progeny; Thanatos, the
death instinct which seeks Nirvana (literally "blowout,"
i.e., the extinguishing of self-awareness) as a goal and
which perpetuates martyrdom in the species.

Tantra doctrine and European philosophy of the
Nietzschean type recognize birth, love and death as
significant events forming a trinity of unparalleled
sensory experience.

Whenever humans have speculated upon the
philosophical implications of the individual journey
from womb to tomb, their conclusions have been
ambivalent.

Concerning birth, we might remember the pessi-
mistic Greek maxim stating that never to be born, or to
die young, are the only blessings that befall men.
Turning to a purely Western viewpoint, it seems that we

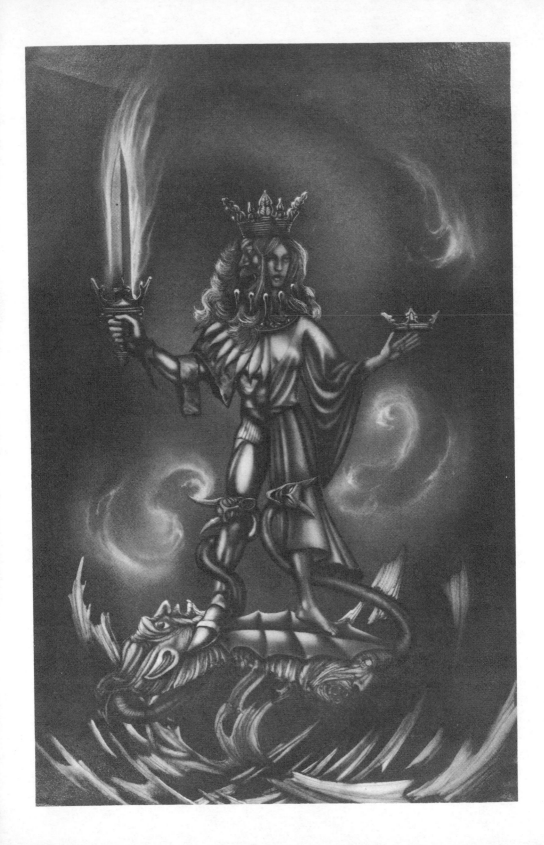

must concur with the psychologist Otto Rank when he designates birth as the first and primary trauma. Genesis, Chapter One, is an allegory of personal birth, the transition from dark, amniotic waters to the blazing light of the environment. "And God said, let there be light; and there was light."

More literature has been produced upon the topic of Eros and erotica than upon any other subject. Eros is a word whose meaning is laden with physical and psychological ambiguities.

At the sexual level, algolagnia is a term covering the range of sadomasochistic feeling associated with Eros. Algolagnia is sexual pleasure aroused by giving or receiving pain. This linkage is inevitable, for we are all a mixture of such tendencies, and to express Eros physically implies both pain and surrender—a surrender of the self to an eternal moment beyond the ego. Many women do not realize that the act of intercourse is as much a surrender for the male as the female. At the moment of orgasm a man sacrifices the essence of his physical being, and this culmination leaves many deeply immersed in a feeling of impending death or "horror vacui."

Eros and Thanatos are twin brothers psychologically, and for the male of the species the two unite even more vividly at the physical level. Extending upwards from the second bone of the neck is a toothlike protuberance called the odontoid process. This "tooth" fits into a cradle in the top bone of the neck called the atlas. (Atlas in Greek mythology held the heavens up, and since heaven is really a state of mind, what better name for the bone which directly supports the skull?) Execution of a man by hanging involves the expert placing of the hangman's knot under the left ear in such a position that the odontoid process is fractured at the end of the drop, rupturing the adjacent spinal cord. This produces a simultaneous ejaculation at the exact moment of the final death convulsion. Eros and

Thanatos transform the gibbet into a nuptial bed and cohabit in a last orgiastic gesture.

The concept of Eros extends beyond the realm of the concrete into that of a universal abstraction of feeling. The Golden Age of the Greeks contrasted Agape or brotherly love with the sexual connotations of Eros. Among the Indo-Aryans, Vedic literature has always differentiated between Kama (lust) and Prem, which suggests love of an intrinsically spiritual nature. Certain schools of thought, peculiar to both civilizations, have always advocated an agamic existence as the ideal state for a select few. Such a sexless existence can only be borne comfortably by those born with hormonal deficiencies genetically programmed. Alternatively, recent research indicates that meditation in caves and catacombs, subjecting the meditator to light deprivation, effectively permits the pineal gland to secrete a substance which dries up and shrinks the gonads.

In general, however, Eros is a means to spiritual experience and not an antagonist. After all, the word "spiritual" etymologically gives rise to "spirited" and concepts like "high spirited."

However much some are prone to ignore the physical manifestations of Eros, they cannot escape confrontation with the Tanric technique of commencing with Kama and converting it into Prem. The pedagogue of English occultists, Aleister Crowley, brilliantly elucidates the method in his book *Magick in Theory and Practice*. The adept is instructed to visualize the interior of his skull as the universal Yoni, and to cultivate the sensation that his spine is an erect lingam ever striving for the union of eternity. Kundalini arousal is a spinal cord ejaculation into the chalice of the skull, using as semen cerebral spinal fluid.

Thanatos has achieved its own place of literary eminence among the Tibetans and Egyptians. Their respective tomes of the dead represent the sum total of human necrology.

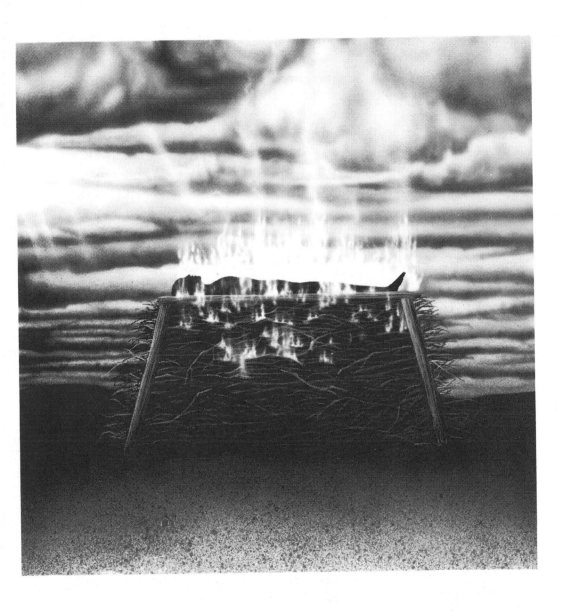

Asia has always possessed a more mature attitude concerning death than that prevalent in the West, for long acquaintance with death as a fundamental reality produces an inherent emotional immunity which Occidental people lack.

One of the most aesthetic memories of my life concerns the cremation of a wealthy Hindu in a Bombay park. The eldest son ignited the ghee, which had been placed in the mouth of his father's flower-strewn body, and having thus witnessed the consecration of the corpse into the purifying embrace of Agni, we sat under an azure sky and chatted hours away while the funeral bier plumed perfumed smoke.

Oriental indifference to death is perhaps best exemplified by the Jain priest of "Muni" who, upon reaching old age and realizing his inability to contribute any longer to his community, retreats into the wilderness and fasts unto death. A tradition also exists among the initiated that some men, upon achieving realization, immediately commit suicide, transforming Samadhi into Maha-samadhi. To paraphrase Castaneda's favored slogan, "Death is the biggest kick of them all—that's why they save it till last."

But what of Eros and Thanatos together? It is now that my personal philosophy intrudes, for I look upon life as a fading fruit unless it contains the vital element of love or "Shakti" (literally "shaking" with aroused energy) firing the Nadis or nervous system. I eternally dwell in the blood shafts of a setting sun whose ember glow pervades everything I see and reveals the death intertwined in life and my own being. In such a seemingly schizophrenic thought there is great beauty, for the antithesis of any given thing confers meaning upon it. Light is insignificant without darkness, and life is meaningless without death.

To love is to go beyond one's own ego, to transcend the failings of the self and lose self-awareness in the contemplation of an imagined ideal person or cause that is really the self in disguise. This is very much like dying, for in

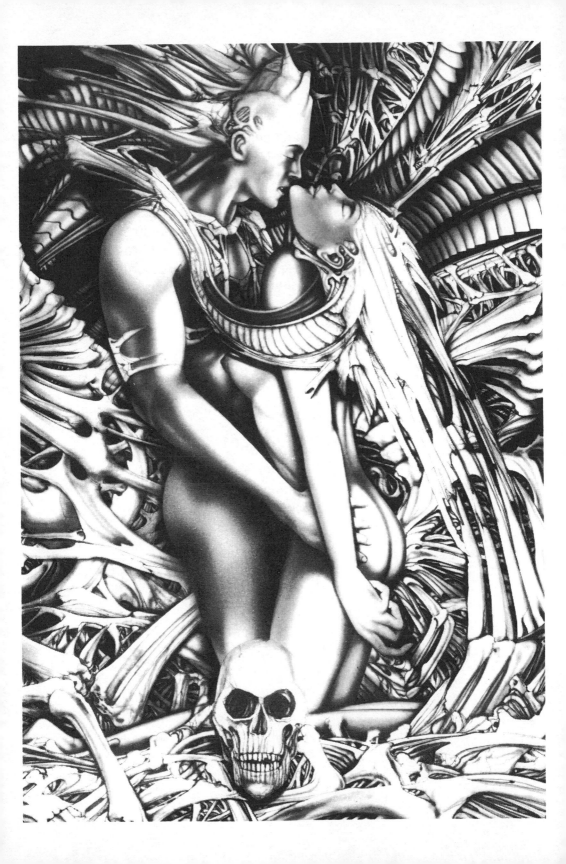

death we are also self-transcendent. Such feelings impel others, philosophically, toward Thanatos, which in Asian tradition is the true God men seek. Thanatos is really the manifest God of East and West, whether we call the son Krishna or Christ, for death is the final surrender. Like a spasm of love it is a thrust out from the self; a giving of body and mind to a paradoxical state of oblivious consciousness.

Thanatos is a drug called nepenthe. Thanatos performs a Procrustean ritual. Birth and death become the only significant events in life, and love is the tension point stretched across the abyss between them.

Tantra, Modern Witchcraft and Psychedelic Drugs

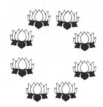

THE EMERGENCE OF modern witchcraft in England and America is an atavistic resurgence of staggering proportions. Any successful system presupposes a need, and I would suggest that modern witchcraft is the Tantra of Western man emerging in the twentieth century to quench his thirst for the vigorous and vital in the inner life.

Startling similarities between Tantra and modern witchcraft indicate that the primal layers of the unconscious, in East and West, seek satisfaction in an earth cult which is matriarchal and feministic. These common features are couched in the symbolical language of myth and allegory, which is a form of communication beyond time, history, science and logic.

Tantra centers around Sahkti as the active feminine pole responsible for dynamic manifestation. This is the direct equivalent of the "Great Mother Goddess" which is the focal point for worship by members of the Wicca.

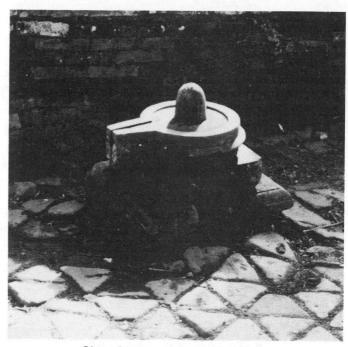

Shiva Lingam showing Yoni base.
Changunarayan Temple, Nepal.

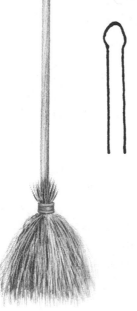

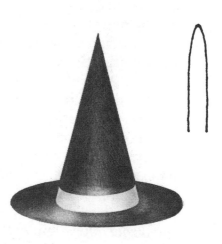

Chakra Puja, or the circle of worshipers, alternating male and female, is the paradigm of the coven, with an emphasis upon ritual nudity prominent in both groups. The purpose of a circle (in itself a womb or feminine symbol) is to enclose and entrap the psychic (pranic) energies exuded by the naked, living flesh of the participants. As their sexual-emotional excitement increases, more radiation or "steam" is produced for occult use. This energy forms a "cone of power" over the group and is similar to the whirling vortex of psychic force released during copulation.

At the risk of appearing trite or simplistic, the resemblance between the Shiva Linga (the central phallic symbol of Tantra) and the witch's broomstick and cone hat must be pointed out.

The broomstick, at unconscious levels, is an elongated Shiva Linga or penis. From time immemorial the broom has been the symbol of woman as dominator and matron of the house, and indeed the very broom plant is itself a diuretic drug, flushing the system of excess fluids and acting as a genito-urinary tract stimulant. Flying, associated with riding the broomstick (masturbation?), is a universal dream motif always indicative, from the analytical viewpoint, of disguised orgasmic experience.

If the broomstick may be described as an "elongated" Shiva Linga, then the classical cone hat of the witch is a "pointed" Shiva Linga, with the rim representing the vagina (Yoni) base upon which it rests, the peak thrusting skyward in imitation of the "cone of power" raised by the coven or Tantra Chakra Puja.

In the *Gnostica* issue of August 21, 1973, appears a summary of the principles of modern witchcraft by the Grandmaster of the First Wiccan Church of Minnesota. The entire credo could be easily mistaken for a Tantric manifesto several thousand years old. I have just taken the first three items as particularly stunning examples of a transcultural attitude spanning time and diverse civilizations:

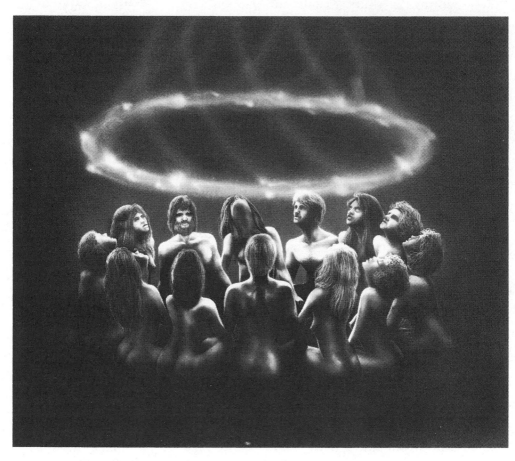

Cone of Power

- Recognition of polarity in all manifestation, including the manifestation of Divinity as Male and Female Forces. [Tantric equivalent is the concept of Shiva-Shakti; Radha-Krishna.]

- Recognition of Divinity manifesting within all life—including the Divinity within Man and Woman. [An answering echo is found in the mantric affirmation, "Ham Sa," "Sa Ham"; "He I am, I am He."]

- Recognition of the Feminine as the "flower" of the race—that woman incarnates beauty and fruitfulness, and through her we reach fulfillment. This has several corollaries:

  a) that woman as the flower is the queen. She must be in the light, as the natural flower needs sunshine, in order to bear and transmit the fruits of love, magick, and human endeavor;

  b) that woman becomes the criterion or our work—that is: as woman is the flower of the race, its adornment, so can our work be measured in terms of its adornment to woman. Simply stated, the goal of all work is seen as beauty, fruitfulness, fulfillment;

  c) that our attitude toward woman is our attitude toward the race and toward life itself. If we limit her creativity, we make the race suffer. If we glorify her, we glorify the race. When we protect her health, we protect the health of the race. When we love woman, we love the race;

  d) that it is Divinity as feminine, our Goddess, who is our Queen. We set her above us, not as a ruler, but as one we adore—who expresses our highest ideals of beauty and life fulfilled;

  e) that it is our rule that that woman who fills the

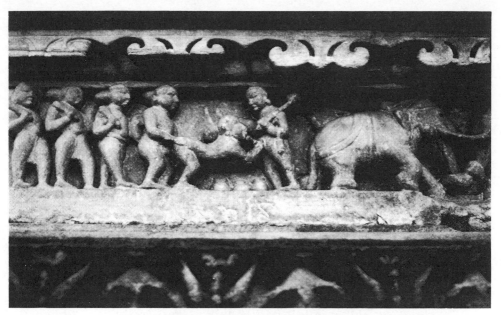

Vishvanath Temple, Khajuraho.

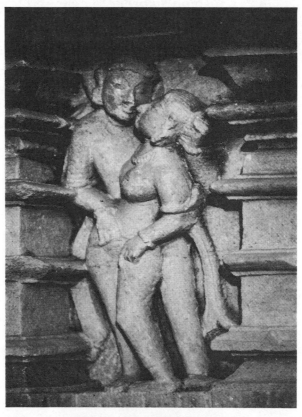

Lakshmana Temple, Khajuraho.

role of High Priestess in our covens, or as our Great Queen, must express the feminine at its fullness—and thus it is that a woman who passes her time of fruitfulness must retire in favor of a younger woman;

f) that there is in that essence of femininity, woman's monthly cycle, the source of our symbolic understanding of the Feminine Force in nature. Thus, her symbol is the Moon, and we say that our Goddess is the Earth Mother, and her daughter (who is also herself) is the Moon Goddess, and behind her is the Great Mother, life itself.

The above axioms* of the contemporary witchcult restate the Tantric doctrine of Shakti incarnate into a body which is a veritable castle of Brahman. She is worshiped through actual or imagined intercourse as an act of submission to the goddess principle of being.

Modern witchcraft, as would be suspected, is replete with a magical technology; i.e., the doctrine that changes can be made to occur in conformity with the will through "subtle" or "non-physical" agencies. One aspect of Tantra also deals with activation of magical forces through Mantra (sound employed as in spells, charms, invocations and evocations) and Yantra (drawing of geometrical shapes and diagrams which act as "transistor" circuits or channels conducting psychic essences).

A special magical potency attributed to menstruation and menstrual fluid is also common to both schools. The Tantric initiate values the menses of his Shakti as a psychically efficacious time for certain practices of occultism.

---

*It should be remembered that these principles pertain to a "magical religion," and reflect the "magical viewpoint" that is its keynote. In other words it is the *inner vision* that is being directed to perceive woman as "the flower of the race" and it is part of the magical ritual that we should "glorify her." These principles should not be used to justify discriminatory practices, whether apparently protective or glorifying.

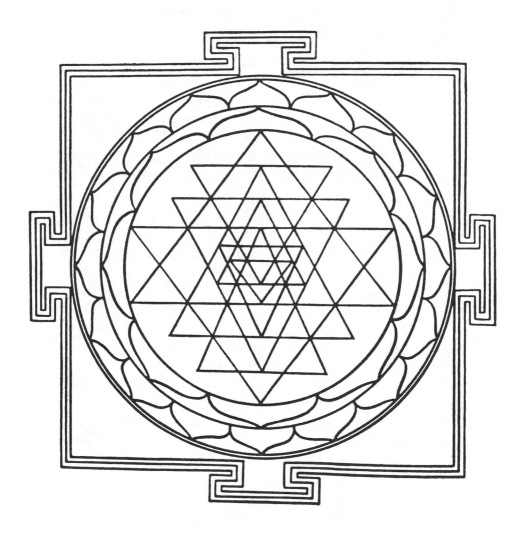

Sri Yantra

In passing it should be mentioned that secretions and trance states obtained as a result of ritual oral intercourse are responsible for the popular growth of the Vampire legend in medieval Europe. This theory, mentioned by the occult research writer Francis King *(Sexuality, Magic, and Perversion),* has merit as revealing the hidden key to the sado-masochistic and orgiastic overtones of the Vampire prototype so exciting to our Victorian ancestors. It also contains the Tantric mystery of how one human can live on the "blood" of another.

The comments I have made comparing Tantra and witchcraft are incomplete, fragmentary and only intended to point the way for further research. It should be noted that I am not suggesting categorically that a direct relationship exists between Tantra and the evolution of today's witchcraft as a formal and legal (at least in the United States) mode of religious worship; however, it is not impossible that such a lineage could be traced, for Tantra is the antecedent spiritual culture of Hinduism, Yoga, Samkhya and the four other classical schools of Hindu philosophy, and has exerted a profound influence on Buddhism as well.

Paramapansa Swami Satyananda Saraswati, the great Tantric Guru of Monghyr, Bihar State, North India, has stated in his book *Tantra Yoga Panorama,* "Six thousand years ago almost two thirds of the human population in Mexico, North America, in France, Egypt, the Middle East, Afghanistan, India, Ceylon, Thailand, Tibet, China, Japan and many other lands practised this science."

PSYCHEDELIC DRUGS: *EAST AND WEST*

In closing this chapter, a few comments about mind expansion are appropriate. The use of psychedelic substances has been traditional in some Tantric and Yoga schools for several thousand years. However, the methods and circumstances under which they are utilized differ greatly from those in contemporary Western practices of "tripping." Aldous Huxley even went so far as to suggest that the practices of Yoga (Tantra) were developed as compensation for loss of access to hallucinogenic mushrooms ("Soma") by the Aryans when they migrated into the Indus Valley.

Patanjali lists "Aushadhi," or drugs, as one of the legitimate means by which Samadhi is attained. Note well the following pointed remarks from Swamihi Satyananda's *Tantra of Kundalini Yoga:*

> The fourth method of awakening according to Yoga is through herbs. In Sanskrit, the word is *aushadhi* but it should not mean drugs. Through herbs either the partial or the fuller awakening can be brought about. Either the awakening of IDA or PINGALA or a awakening of SUSHUMNA which means the entire, total wakening can be brought about. That is known as AUSHADHI but it is also said that the herbs which should be used to awaken this potentiality, or this life in man should be understood or should be got only through the GURU, not without a GURU. Because there are certain herbs that awaken IDA and there are others that can awaken PINGALA only; and there are those that can even suppress both of these two so that you can go to the mental asylum very quickly! So the question of AUSHADHI or the herbal awakening is a very risky, quick but unreliable method. *It should only be got from one who is a very reliable person and who knows the science very well.*

Besides the opium, magic mushrooms and hashish known to Western pharmacology, other psychotomimetics are prepared from plants indigenous to India and relatively unfamiliar in the Occident. To such plants or herbs are attributed pranic energies which will temporarily arouse Kundalini and cause the chakras to blossom. They may be described as "spiritual abortifacents," in some cases producing premature psychic experiences which may result (for the untrained individual) in as many survival problems as the physical counterpart of premature birth for the infant.

The problem lies not in achieving Kundalini arousal (by drugs or any method) but rather in how to handle, control and direct the resultant force. Again quoting Swamiji Satyananda *(Tantra of Kundaline Yoga):*

> Those who are eager to awaken the Chakras should not do anything in a hurry or should not be anxious. They should set apart 12 years of their life for this purpose. I do not mean that in one or three years it cannot be done. Everything can be done in one month also. Awakening can take place in one month, three months, in one day, even the Guru can give you awakening but you can not hold it. You can not sustain it, if it is awakening. With a weak mind which can not sustain a little bit of cheerfulness, a little bit of excitement, which can not sustain the death of a man or the separation of husband and wife, how can it sustain that terrible force of the flow of SHAKTI? Therefore, 12 years are not for the awakening, twelve years are to prepare yourself to hold the awakening. "When you live with a GURU and prepare your mind, soul and heart, the body and nerves and the glands, the actions, your reactions, your opinions and each and every part of your personality is seasoned, is shaped. For that twelve years are required because the human being takes a long time to change himself. Whereas the awakening of the CHAKRAS, I would say, is not a matter of a long time and it can take place anytime.

The difference between the Yogin's culminating Sadhana or spiritual practice with psychedelic substances and the Western student's lazily short-cutting by chemical "mind-blowing" are considerable. These distinctions may be enumerated as follows:

- Indiscriminate use of consciousness-expanding drugs without prior mental training and the absolute physical discipline imparted by years of Hatha and Raja Kriya is equivalent to dynamiting open the door to a treasure vault (the unconscious mind) and discovering the blast has destroyed half the treasure plus irreparably damaging the door so that it cannot easily be shut at will.

• The karmic basis of life is that a price is exacted for everything, including illumination. The Yogi or Tantrist pays his karma through years of practice and discipline well before ever opening the mind with a psychedelic drug. Under such circumstances the initiate in the Eastern tradition achieves realization without deleterious side effects. On the contrary, most Westerners dropping "acid" or other such substances risk paying a karmic debt after the experience with depression, inability to cope, de-realization, depersonalization, psychological malaise, and in some cases precipitation of latent schizophrenia or recurrent psychotic episodes.

• Theoretically, the quality of the subjective nature of the drug experience may differ radically between the Yogin and the average Occidental. Diet control coupled with certain very powerful internal cleansing techniques peculiar to advanced phases of Hatha Yoga may so thoroughly rinse the major cavities of the body (sinuses, stomach, large and small intestine, uro-genital system) that the phlegm, mucus and poisons, encouraging deleterious micro-organisms and metabolites in the blood stream, are removed.

　　The subjective experience of the the Eastern meditator is the result of biochemical changes wrought in a pure blood stream carrying the ingested drug through the brain. For others, their subjective state is compounded of the drug mixed with the poisonous metabolites of their normally "dirty" blood stream filtering through the brain tissue. An apt comparison would be the difference between tasting soup made from a mud puddle and a broth created from clear, bubbling spring water.

Shank Prakshalana is one example of a popular internal cleansing method used in North Indian Tantric schools. Shank Prakshalana totally flushes out the gastro-intestinal tract by passing several gallons of saline solution from the mouth through the numerous convolutions of the intestinal tract and out through the anus. The passage and expulsion of the fluid is assisted by special Asanas or postures which squeeze the stomach and wring out the gut. At initiation Indian hemp or bhang (marijuana) is sometimes added to the Shank Prakshalana water, thus producing trance consciousness as the cleansing procedure deepens.

From the Tantric viewpoint drug-induced ecstasy is a legitimate device which may sometimes be employed at a certain phase of training to facilitate the unlocking of the universe contained in the skull. The drug experience for the trained disciple is invariably clear, always under control and positive in terms of reintegrating the practitioner—never disintegrating him.

Finally we may sum up by noting that Tantra eschews "no-thing" that may aid man to become "real-ized." Certainly the sexual impulse is a valuable tool for most aspirants, and mind-expanding drugs under special guidance may assist others. Although the major topic of this book has been sex magic and Tantric sexual practices, it must not be assumed that the whole of Tantra is concerned with these aspects. Tantra is the life science concerned with producing true individuals. The literal meaning of the word "individual" is "un-divided" or "in-divisible." What higher goal could be sought than to become truly in-dividual?

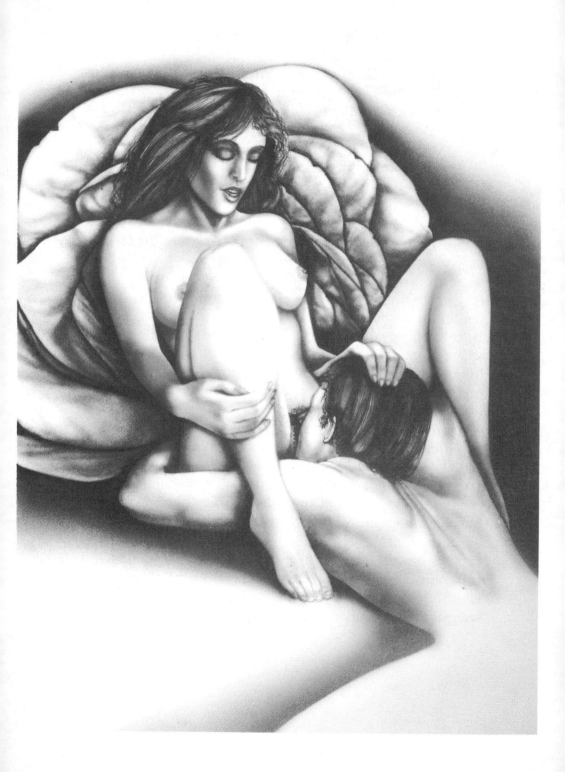

Afterword
Love and Romance
by
Carl Llewellyn Weschcke

WHERE DO LOVE and romance come into the picture? Let's ask ourselves what romance does to us that we yearn so for it. And what is it we feel when we are in love that is so important?

In love, we are overcome with *awareness* of the beloved person: in everything we do, we think of him or her. And "think" isn't the right word—for it is rather that we are completely occupied with feelings for the beloved person, and we want to bring those feelings into our every moment of awareness.

When we are in love, we glow! We're more alive, and we know it and other people know it. We *love* love, and we *adore* lovers.

Romance is a kind of ritual which recognizes the special awareness that comes with being in love—which expresses that awareness and extends into behavioral patterns that anthropologists call "courtship rites." We bring our beloved flowers and other gifts; we clean and arrange our apartments to prepare for him or her; we dress with care and awareness of the attractive powers of our costume; we arrange special foods and entertainment; and so on. In short, we create an *environment* that favors love, and has a direction to it that should—after a while—lead to the consummation of that love.

Now that we've read this book, we should also perceive that through this ritual of romance we are building erotic tension and actually acting in a way which, in a religious situation, is described as "worship." When we are in love, we truly do worship our beloved, and in that person we are finding the highest expression of Life as we can know it. We want to be with our beloved all the time, and we can perceive no greater joy than union with her or him.

Remember what it is like to be in love, and realize that it is the Life Force at its fullest seeking fulfillment. It is the biology of reproduction programming the behavior of two people to carry out not merely "the physical act of sex" but to accomplish it with the total focus of all psychic and spiritual energies of two people to enable the incarnation of a third person whose destiny is intertwined with theirs.

It's the God and Goddess within, worshiping each other, and uniting to produce a new physical body perfectly suited to the incarnating soul. What higher act of magick do we normally experience than this?

In Tantra we re-capture that union of God and Goddess, and we do it with awareness of the Deity within each and the other. Perhaps some of us are older, and the first flush of first love has long since departed. Can "philosophic appreciation" of the Tantric view of life raise the richness of body and psychic heat we experienced in our first love?

It cannot, unless we add to it the elements found in Romance and the rites of courtship. Much of Tantra can be seen in the externals of ritual—rituals which combine symbolism meaningful to the culture of the participants with actions that produce the natural build-up of energies we've just described.

Romance, like Magick, involves the creation of a special

environment, an *atmosphere,* and ritual actions focus the inner awareness, to *arouse the Divine Life Force within.*

In the "Tantric Weekend" that follows, you will see an example of this. It is not a ritual that must be followed to the letter, but is offered only as an example or as a framework around which you may compose your own. The point to remember is that you are preparing a *drama* in which you are acting out the deepest and most powerful programming of your entire genetic system, and you are giving it a new focus: creating a *Magical Child* that is your own spiritual growth, or that may be anything else you magically desire.

You may better appreciate it as *worship.* Give it all the attention that you would, knowing you are preparing a place for God and Goddess.

Your Temple, your Priestly Robes, your Sacraments, and your Ritual Adorations are all focused on the glory of the Goddess and the God—the Divine Manifestation of Feminine and Masculine Life Force, the *Yin/Yang* of Creation. You can bring into play your perception of these Forces as they seek expression in your consciousness as various powerful Archetypes; you can dress yourselves in dramatic "assumption" of these God- or Goddess-images; you can—if you dare—arouse the deepest roots of your sexual drives with the use of *fetish and fantasy.*

Always prolong the "foreplay"—the build-up. The "Tantric Weekend" states that your goal is to raise the Life Force within to *fever pitch* and still keep it in bounds, use it to increase your awareness and perception. Add richness to your appreciation of your partner with the perception that he/she is "God and Goddess alive" at the same time that he/she is "soul sharing your life."

Love and Lust are both four letter words. Together they add up to eight letters, like the word "Marriage." That's what our ritual is accomplishing: marriage is a true union (having little to do with the legal institution by the same name) of Male and Female. We can limit our conception of that to the union of Man and Woman, or extend it to that of the most dynamic powers in the Universe. In Tantra, we know that we are Divine, and in our union the Creative Forces are raised and can bring into manifestation our *Magical Child.*

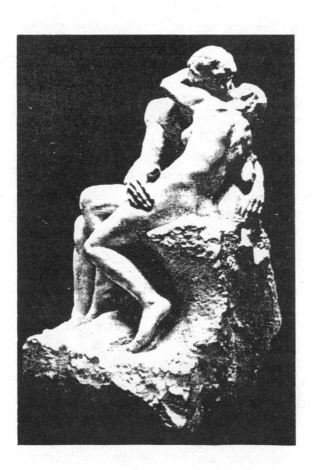

A Tantric Weekend
by
Donald Michael Kraig

IT HAS BEEN noted by many people that the passion quickly leaves the relationship of married or monogamous lovers. This passion is a necessity for the practice of Tantra, and the loss of passion may be the reason why some couples have little success with Tantra.

However, it does not have to be that way. Monogamous and married couples are the *ideal* Tantric partners. The familiarity a person has with his or her partner can help them in their Tantric practices. Even more important, Tantra can actually enhance their relationship so that the love and passion need never leave it. Tantra is not only a boon for couples today, but is rapidly becoming a necessity.

Here are two ways by which Tantra can improve relationships. First, the practice of Tantra can bring ecstatic sexual experiences. However, Tantra is *more* than just sex—it is a way of life. The life of a Tantric is one of discovery of the ecstatic experience in *everyday* life. This is more than just "stopping to smell the roses," it is experiencing the roses as a joyous gift from the Divine to you.

Passion is important in all aspects of life. The passionate practice of Tantra can bring on the goal of true yoga: Nirvana (also known as Samadhi), enlightenment, and cosmic consciousness. Part of Nirvana, the experience of unity with the universe, is the awareness that everything is special, whether it is seeing a flower for the first time or making love with your mate for the ten-thousandth time. Most people do not see this "specialness" in everything. A Tantric does.

The mystic Georges Gurdjieff had the same notion, saying that most people were asleep, not even paying attention to what was going on around them. For example, do you remember what items were in the windows of the stores you passed when you last went by them, or were you asleep? Chances are that although you functioned as if you were awake, a major part of your sensory apparatus was turned off or "asleep." A goal of Tantra is to turn you on to the world, to wake you from your sleep and bring passion to all aspects of your life.

The following weekend experience is for those who want to awake to the greater universe. It will deepen your experience of life. It will also help you to deepen the relationship with your love partner. In the world today, many people take this most important relationship either not seriously enough or too seriously. They don't pay enough attention to it, or take it so seriously that much of the spontaneity and fun has gone out of it. This Tantric Weekend will help to bring out a deeper bond in your relationship, while at the same time make it more fun.

A second way by which Tantra can enhance a relationship is by combating a demon that stalks most realtionships. This terrible demon, known for its green eyes, has not only destroyed many relationships, but has also left pain, anger, hatred and violence in its wake. This demon's name: jealousy.

Jealousy has many causes, but perhaps the two most important ones are poor self-image and fear. Actually, these two are interrelated. For example, if a woman has a poor self-image and sees her lover talking with another woman, she may become afraid that her partner will find the new woman more exciting. She may fear that her partner will leave her for the new woman. Anger and bitterness may follow. This can damage the relationship even if the partner has no desire to leave the woman. Men, for same reasons, may feel jealousy if they see their love partner talking to another man.

Many times the strength of love in a relationship can barely hold sway over the demon jealousy. Too frequently, jealousy wins and the relationship deteriorates or ends. There is a way to defeat this demon and empower a relationship so much that jealousy is permanently prevented from destroying the realtionship. It is the way of Tantra.

The following Tantric Weekend willl help you on the path to overcoming jealousy and enhancing your relationship to a level you may have not thought possible. It will develop your trust in your partner to a level far beyond anything you might imagine. At the same time it will open your senses to this world. In fact, it will help open your senses to a degree where everything becomes a sacrament, and daily living becomes a spiritual and magickal ritual.

In the past, Tantric devotees were expected to give up all of their possessions, quit work, and beg for shelter and a few scraps of food. This may have been fine for ancient India, but it is not practical for most of us in the West today. Thus, the training in this Tantric Weekend is designed to be perfect for Westerners. It would begin Friday after work or school and end on Sunday evening. Before going on, decide now: is your relationship worth one weekend? Is your spiritual growth worth two days and three nights?

If so, read over the directions for this Tantric Weekend together. Plan it out together and agree to go along with the ideas presented here. Also, agree that either of you may choose to end the weekend experience at anytime, but that if this occurs you will repeat it in the future.

A final thought: chances are you will have never experienced the type of sex as described in the Tantric Weekend. It is not goal (i.e. orgasm) oriented. Rather, it focuses on the sensuality of joy, fun and non-goal oriented sexual expression. The long buildup to the final sexual release on Sunday evening can lead to a senses shattering experience of release and unity with the universe. This is true Nirvana.

Preparations

Many people have a feeling that for sex to be "right" it must be spontaneous. In Tantra it is believed that you can prepare for sex and still allow the actual sexual experience to be free and spontaneous. In other words, there can be freedom within a structure. Thus, preparing for a special weekend of sexuality should bring happiness into your life rather than the feeling that spontaneity will be missing. In fact, you will find even more spontaneity within this weekend structure.

Your first preparation should be to plan for your Tantric Weekend well in advance. If possible, take a vacation for this weekend. It doesn't have to be far or to an expensive place, just someplace new and different. If it is near a large park, forest, lake or ocean, so much the better. Plan this out together.

If you have children, get someone to take care of them for your weekend. Tell the sitters you will exchange the favor for them and watch their children for a whole weekend in the future. Tell people you will be out of town (even if you're not leaving) so they won't try to call you on the telephone. Plan a weekend where you and your love partner can be alone.

Next, plan to turn your hotel or motel room, or your house or apartment, into a place for Tantra. This will include cleaning it up if necessary. Get some candles for light and incense for smell. Bring in some foods which can be easily prepared without trouble. Fruits, juices, wines (drunk in small amounts only), various breads and rolls, nuts, small sweets, cheeses, etc. are perfect for this purpose.

You will also want to prepare yourselves for this Tantric Weekend. Splurge a bit. After all, your relationship is worth it! Women should obtain some quality costume make-up and lots of decorative jewelry. Why not get some erotic clothes, too? This does not necessarily mean garter belts

127

and high heels. Rather, a loose, possibly semi-transparent garment that shows off your curves would be perfect. Men can get loose drawstring pants, large shirts and jewelry. You probably know what your partner likes. If not, ask him or her.

Finally, get some sensuality toys. By this I don't mean the devices many people think of as sex toys. Instead, focus on sensuality and all of the senses, not just sex. Include perhaps a fur glove and a feather for gently stroking the skin of your partner. Also include some scented oils to massage into the skin. Perhaps some extra gauzy pieces of material to wrap around each other and even some body paints (paints which will come off the skin in the shower or bath). Get everything you would like to try. Also, get a blindfold. Be sure to read the instructions for the Tantric Weekend *before* starting. Make sure that there is nothing else you need to plan or do before actually moving onto the next section.

Friday Evening

The children are away, the phone is off the hook, or you are in your vacation retreat. Chances are you are tired from your day's work and/or travel. Before going on to the next step, you should begin to relax. One of you can begin decorating the place with the candles and incense while the other person takes a leisurely warm bath in water scented with perfume, oils or bath salts. Let your cares fade away. When the first person leaves the tub, he or she can finish decorating and preparing the area while the partner takes a bath. When bathing and preparations are finished you should together light the incense and candles, then turn out any electric lights. Let the magick begin!

Dinner

By now you should both have on your special lounging clothes. This weekend you will not feed yourself. Rather, your partner will feed you whenever you are hungry. Start with one partner feeding the other. If you are feeding a man, realize that this man is also a manifestation of that aspect of Divinity we call God. Tell him you love him. Similarly, if you are feeding a woman partner, realize that she is a manifestation of that aspect of Divinity we call Goddess. As you feed her tell her you love her. When the first person being fed is no longer hungry (not "stuffed to the gills," just no longer hungry), change roles.

Play! Tease each other. Laugh. But remember, there is a point where teasing is no longer fun or funny. Be aware of this point by being aware of your partner's moods.

IMPORTANT: During this entire Tantric Weekend you should only discuss the here-and-now. Do not discuss something which happened a year ago, or even yesterday. Do not talk about anything further in the future than this weekend. Also, don't discuss what's on TV or what the football team is doing or how the kids are.

So what should you talk about? Talk about yourselves. Tell your partner how you like his laugh or the sparkle in her eye. Tell her about the sweetness of the fruit or that tartness of the cheddar cheese. Compliment each other, but make it real—if you don't believe it, your partner won't believe it either!

Next, play some music and dance with each other. The music should be slow and without words so you can concentrate on each other, not on the vocalist. If you can't dance, don't worry about it. Just hold each other and sway in time to the music.

In all of this, take your time! There is no rush, no one to bother you. By now it should be after nine or ten in the evening. Your dancing, swaying and touching one another should have been arousing. Blow out all of the candles except for a few in the bedroom. Make sure that there is no way they could tip over and start a fire. Have some water, juice, or wine (or two or all three of them) by the bed. Go to bed *still in your lounging clothes.*

Now, realize that you are in the same bed with a God

or Goddess—not just your partner, but with Divinity itself! Caress your partner. Ask him or her if she or he likes what you are doing. Ask them if they want it firmer or gentler. Caress and kiss each other as much as you like, but keep your clothes on! If either partner is about to have an orgasm, tell your partner to stop the caresses. You should both become incredibly aroused, but not have an orgasm. You may caress your partner over their clothes, you may also reach under their clothes, but do not remove any clothes.

When the tension reaches a peak, stop! Relax for a few moments. Concentrate on calming your breath. Let it return to normal. Then repeat this process. After reaching this pre-orgasmic peak at least two times, and at the most, five times, stretch out on the bed, facing each other, the man on his left side and the woman on her right. Hug each other, and *breathe at opposite times.* That is, when one partner breathes in, the other should exhale, and vice-versa. Continue this breathing until your breathing returns to normal or until you fall asleep. If your breathing has returned to normal and you have not fallen asleep, you may wish to change your position to become more comfortable and go to sleep. Remember, if you talk, discuss the here and now.

Saturday

After you awake, feed each other, as you did the night before. Take your time, laugh, have fun, and keep your talk to the here and now.

Now, one partner should be blindfolded. A large piece of cloth will do, and if the person can see through it he or she can just shut their eyes. The partner without the blindfold should be a guide to the blindfolded person. Guide them around the rooms and have them touch different objects. Have them describe the object. Is it cold? Hard? Wet? Dry? Ask questions about it. Take the person outside, too. Ask them what they hear. Ask them what they smell. Guide them around the park or beach or lake or just around the block. Have the blindfolded person hold your forearm when you walk. You are doing two things: first, you are helping them to open up their senses. Most of our sensory input comes through the eyes. By eliminating this sense, our other senses become more open and alive. The blindfolded person will experience things never before consciously experienced. Second, the person who is blindfolded must also have perfect trust in you. This trust will grow as he or she realizes that you are not going to walk them off a cliff or even have them trip over a twig. This trust will help to empower your relationship.

After you have been doing this for about two hours, it will be time to go back to your Weekend hideaway. Remove the blindfold and start walking back. But as you walk back, ask the previously blindfolded person sense oriented questions. Ask him or her what is smelled, what is heard, what is felt. Ask them to describe everything. Also ask the person to describe the different shades of blue or red or green that the person sees. In this way, you are helping the person to keep open those senses as well as make vision more aware.

When you reach your Tantric Weekend home, share your midday meal as before. Then, repeat the blindfold sense opening and trust building, but the partners should reverse their roles. Upon returning, again share a meal in the manner already described.

Saturday Night
After the meal, it is time once again to take a bath, only this time, take the bath together. Laugh. Play. Use the body paints. Arouse each other. Did you remember to burn incense and light the bathroom with candles only? Now, dry each other off with gentle strokes.

Dress in your special, comfortable garments and go to the bed. Make this night a repeat of the previous night, only on a higher level. After you have aroused yourselves two times, slowly, sensually, remove each other's clothing, one

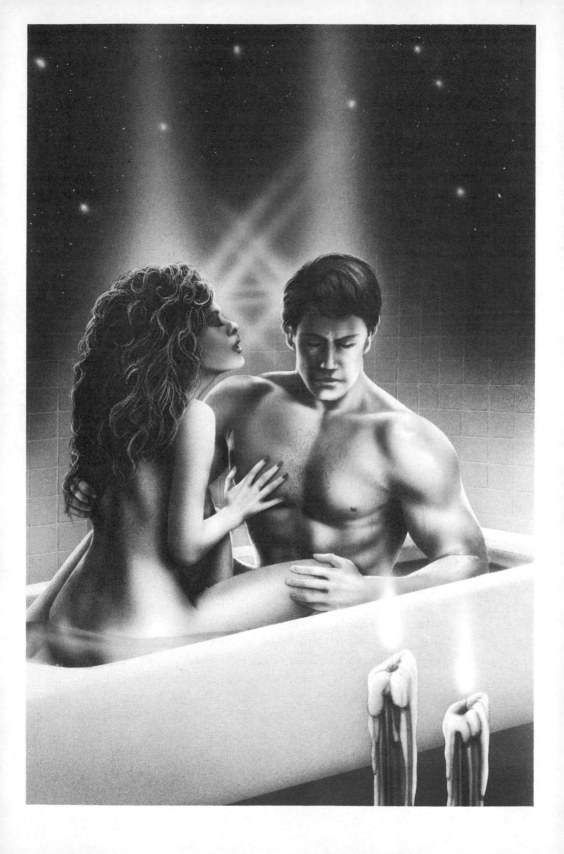

piece at a time. Caress each other, laugh, love one another. Continue until you are both nude, although body jewelry, make-up, oils and scents are appropriate to leave on. Continue the build-up relaxation loving as in the night before. Use some of the toys, such as the fur glove and feather to caress each other. At a loss for originality? Try to find the most sensitive part of your partner's body without your partner saying any words. You partner may moan, writhe, or do nothing; however, your partner should not talk. A sure way to tell if a woman is becoming aroused is by changes in her breathing, increased vaginal lubrication, skin flushing, aroused nipples and writhing motions. In the male, besides an increasingly firm erection, his nipples may become erect, his breathing may change, there may be skin flushing, writhing, and the appearance of lubricating fluid at the tip of the phallus. Do not have intercourse and do not have orgasms.

After reaching the pre-orgasmic peak and relaxing several times, again lay on your sides and do the breathing at opposite times as on the previous night. Similarly, allow yourselves to drift to sleep.

Sunday

Rise and feed each other as before.

Sit down on the floor, or on the bed, so that your backs support each other, that is, you are leaning against each other, back-to-back. Start out by taking turns describing things you like about yourself. Do you like your laugh, your thighs, your breasts, your sense-of-humor? Say so. Take your time and be honest. Then take turns describing what you like about your partner. Again, be honest.

Don't be surprised if you find your partner likes something which you are not particularly fond of. Also, because you are back-to-back, you are actually within each other's aura. Just because you cannot see your partner does not mean you will not be able to pick up on your partner's feelings. In fact, because you are not looking at your partner, it may even be easier to sense your partner's feelings. You will be getting the full impact of their emotions without your attempting to interpret it through your vision (which is only now starting to see everything as the result of yesterday's exercises).

Why do this? So you can come to understand the true depth to which your partner cares about you and loves you, to help you remove your doubts and fears which keep you from having as fulfilling a relationship as you want and need.

When you have finished this exercise (and you can take as long as you like), go to the bed (or use the floor), and begin working on arousing each other. When you reach a peak, stop, but instead of lying on your sides, lay next to each other with one person's head next to the other person's feet and vice-versa. Your right sides should be touching. Place your right hands over the genitals of your partner. Just rest them there. Do the breathing at opposite times as before. When you have relaxed and your arousal has subsided, again work on arousing each other, but when you reach a pre-orgasmic peak, repeat the above procedure, only this time lie with your left sides touching and your left hands on each other's genitalia. After you have done this at least four times, twice ending up on the left and twice on the right, relax, get dressed, take a walk. Did you notice any feelings of energy at the genitals while you were lying next to each other and breathing? If so, say so. If not, it doesn't matter. When you return from your walk, feed each other lunch.

After the usual slow, leisurely lunch of feeding and teasing each other, again take a bath and play with each other. Caress, tease, arouse, and have a good time. Dry each other off and dress in your comfortable clothes. Retire to the bed.

The man should sit cross legged on the bed, in a half or full lotus if possible. A wall may be used to help support his back. The woman should sit on his lap facing him. Her legs should be around his back. Now begin the breathing at opposite times. However, this time add the following visualization. The man should look at the woman's right eye. As he inhales and she exhales, they should sense a flow of energy coming out of her right eye and into his left eye, the eye into which she is looking. The energy should continue down through his body and as he begins to exhale, visualize the energy flowing out of his phallus, into her vagina, and up through her body. Thus, there is a circle of energy being formed which should be visualized by both partners. As you continue, try to sense the energy. Make the energy physical; make it real.

In fact, the energy is real! It is only that until now you have been unable to detect it. But with the exercises of yesterday and today you should begin to really experience the energy. Let it flow.

When you tire, relax from the position, lay next to one another, and share what you felt. As you do this, begin to caress one another and build up to that intense pre-orgasmic state. Again, do not allow yourselves to reach an orgasm. Instead, repeat the above exercise. Do this procedure at least twice clothed and at least twice wearing no clothes. You should allow yourselves no orgasm and you should not have had the phallus enter the vagina. Actually you may repeat this procedure as many times as you like, but usually four to six times will be the limit. Then relax, take a leisurely walk, and feed each other dinner.

The past hours have been an incredible experience. You have learned increasing trust in your partner and how to open your senses. Your sex without orgasm or intercourse will have opened you up to new awarenesses of your sexual responses. You will have learned about your psychic energy flows. You will also be more relaxed than you have been in several weeks, months or even years. And this has all taken place since Friday night!

But along with this has come another great tension, sexual tension. It has also been building since Friday night.

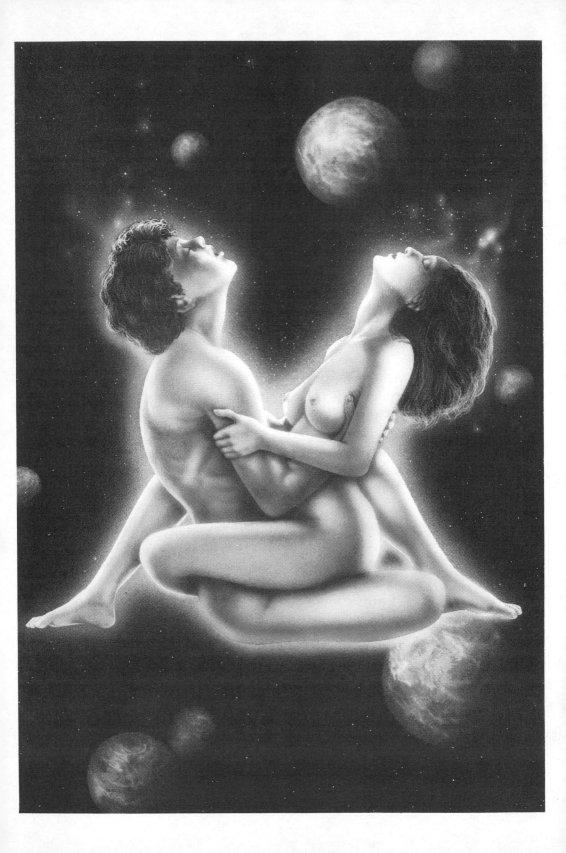

Now comes the time to bring everything together. Even if you do not do the final step as described here, your relationship will end up deeper, more trusting, and closer. You will have empowered yourself with your new knowledge as well as empowering your relationship with a new and greater vitality. The following will help build on that.

Again take a bath together. Excite one another. Play with one another. Then dry each other, dress and retire to the bed. As earlier today, caress, arouse and excite one another until you need to stop before having an orgasm. Then assume the sitting position as earlier and do the opposing breathing and visualization as earlier.

Repeat this procedure, only this time lovingly and playfully remove each other's clothes. At the proper time, assume the sitting position and do the breathing and visualization.

When you have calmed down and relaxed, again repeat the caressing, arousing, playing, teasing and loving. When it reaches a peak, again assume the sitting position, only this time, and for the first time this weekend, one of the partners should insert the phallus in the vagina. Move yourselves around until the phallus is as deeply embedded in the vagina as possible. Then do the opposite breathing with visualization. As this becomes clear, realize that you are making love with the God or Goddess. If an orgasm occurs, fine. If not, that is O.K. too. You may end the session with love-making as you wish.

Do not be surprised if the woman has many orgasms and the man can quickly redevelop an erection after orgasm.

The Tantric Weekend Ends

By this time it should be the middle of the evening. You will have enough time to collect your things and return home or clean up your house. In the past three nights and two days you will have developed and empowered yourself through typical Tantric exercises. You will be able to bring this awareness to your everyday life, making everything you do and everyone you're with more special. Your relationship will continue to deepen and improve. And the sexual aspect of your relationship will reach a new level, perhaps unimagined by you only a few days ago.

    As mentioned at the beginning of this ritual weekend, it may be that one or both of you will decide not to complete the entire weekend as described in the instructions. Remember, Tantra believes in the specialness of everything. Therefore, have no recriminations, no anger, no unhappiness. Enjoy every part of the Tantric Weekend you completed, and also enjoy whatever you did during the rest of the weekend.

    Enjoy life! Enjoy every precious second of it. If you don't complete the Tantric Weekend exactly as in the instructions—fine! If you want to change it around—fine! But at sometime do try to accomplish the Tantric Weekend as described. It can change your life and your relationship for the better. However, if you don't complete it this weekend you can always try it another time.

    Until then, laugh, love, be awake and be happy.

Appendix A:
The Tree of Life[*]

WHEN COMMENCING TO outline and write this book on Magic, it was the firm intention of the writer to elucidate all magical processes as simply and as intelligibly as was both humanly possible and consistent with proper exegetical treatment of a highly difficult and complex subject. Because there has been in the past so much willful obscurity and intentionally misleading matter, it seemed high time to provide a statement which could be utilized once and for all as a clear, definite exposition. The writer hopes that he has kept to this intention throughout, although that is a point of which the reader must be the sole judge. Ambiguity and sometimes deliberate attempts to deceive, through the employment of difficult symbolism and mention of large series of authoritative names, have characterized a number of magical books, thus vitiating whatever value was theirs. There remains to be outlined in this work one secret formula of Practical Magic of such a tremendous nature—shrouded as it always has

* Chapter 16, *The Tree of Life* by Israel Regardie first published by Rider & Co., London, 1932. Rights purchased by Llewellyn Publications 1968. Currently published by Samuel Weiser, Inc.

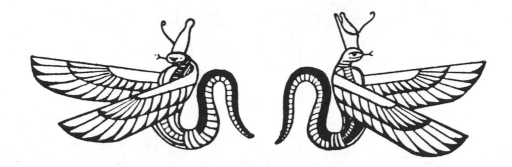

been in the past by the glamour of recondite symbols and hidden by heavy veils—that the writer is doubtful as to whether it would be wise or politic to adhere to his original decision. It might, of course, have been omitted from the general contents, but to render this treatise moderately complete so far as the major, though elementary, aspects of the Higher Magic are concerned, it was necessary to include it in some form. The method of which it is proposed to speak is so puissant a formula of the Magic of Light, and one so liable to indiscriminate abuse and use in Black Magic, that if a conception of its technique and theory is to be presented at all, then the original intent of the writer must be discarded. It will be necessary to resort to the medium of an eloquent symbolism which for centuries has been utilized for the conveyance of these and similar ideas. And the reader must be assured that the symbolism has not been purposely muddled, nor has it been rendered ambiguous, obscure and meaningless. If carefully studied, the terms employed will reveal a consistency and a continuity which will disclose to the right people in a quite accurate manner the processes of its technique.

The Mass of the Holy Ghost! Thus is this particular technique named. It is a unique one in the whole of Magic, for therein are comprehended almost every known form of Theurgic procedure. Simultaneously, it is the quintessence and the synthesis of them all. Among other things it concerns the Magic of Talismans. By this method a living spiritual force is bound into a specific telesmatic substance. Not dead or inert is this telesmata as obtained in the customary ceremonial talismanic evocation; but it is one at once vibrant, dynamic, and containing in germ and potentiality the possibility of all growth and development. In a very special way, it concerns moreover the formula of the Holy Grail. A golden Chalice of spiritual grace is employed, into which the very essence and lifeblood of the Theurgist must be poured for the redemption not of his own soul but that thereby all mankind might be saved.

The Eucharist too is implicit, and the Chalice is used as the communion cup, the hallowed contents of which—thaumaturgic and iridescent; the sacramental wine, in short—must be dedicated and consecrated to the service of the Most High. The Oblation to be consumed with the Eucharist wine is, by this interpretation, the secret essence of both the intoxicated Magician and the supreme God whom he has invoked. In this method also is imputed to a very large degree the alchemical technique, inasmuch as it concerns for the most part the production of the potable Gold, the Stone of the Philosophers, and the Elixir of Life which is Amrita, the Dew of Immortality.

Above all should the reader retain in mind the philosophical formula of the Tetragrammaton which is the method of this Mass. This demonstrates the necessity for a practical acquaintance with the numerical principles of the Holy Qabalah, for the more knowledge one possesses and has systematically classified under the index system of the

Tree of Life, the more meaning and significance attaches itself to the Tetragrammaton formula. In the chapter sketching the magical theory of the universe, the general implications of the sacred Names were briefly explained in those connections. These ideas should be thoroughly assimilated in relation to the Tree. With that understanding the reader should apply his or her powers to the symbolic scheme which now follows.

Illustrating one chapter head in Franz Hartman's *Secret Symbols of the Rosicrucians* is a drawing of a mermaid rising from the sea. To her breasts her hands are held, and there issue therefrom two streams returning into the sea. In explanation of this figure Hartman wrote that "The figure represents the foundation of things and from which all things are born. It is a dual principle of nature; its parents are the Sun and the Moon; it produces water and wine, gold and silver, by the blessing of God. If you torture the Eagle the Lion will become feeble. The 'Eagle's tears' and the 'red blood of the Lion' must meet and mingle. The Eagle and the Lion bathe, eat, and love each other. They will become like the Salamander and become constant in the fire."

In elaboration of the above, the following principles may be postulated. The Y of the sacred Name in this system is called the Red Lion, and the first H is the White Eagle. These two letters are conceived to be the representations of two cosmic principles, two rivers of scarlet blood which pour from the breasts of the mermaid into the sea, two distinct everflowing streams of life and light and love which proceed eternally from Life itself. In them is the power of touching and communing, making new one the other, without any breaking of the subtle confines of the flowing streams, nor any confusion of substance. Mutually complementary and opposite in nature are they; yet in them is grounded the entirety of existence. All alchemical operations according to authority require two major instruments: "one circular, crystalline vessel, justly proportioned to the quality of its contents," or the Cucurbite, and "one theosophic, cabalistically sealed furnace or Athanor."* The Athanor is assigned to the Y, and the Cucurbite is an attribution of the H.

   Now although the pure Gold of which mention was made is a homogeneous substance, one and indivisible, dynamic and pregnant with infinte possibility, nevertheless two separate substances are used in its production. These are named the Serpent or the Blood of the Red Lion, and the Tears or the Gluten of the White Eagle. The Serpent is an attribution of the V of Tetragrammaton, and to the last H of that Name the Gluten is allocated. These two substances are the offspring, as it were, of the Lion and the Eagle. The alchemical instruments aforementioned are to be considered as the storehouses or generators of these two divine principles or swift flowing streams of blood and fire and force, the Athanor being the source or vehicle of the serpent, and the Gluten being housed in the

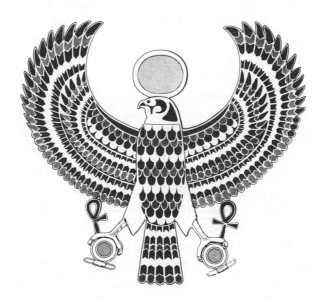

---

* *Amphiteatrum*, H. Khunrath.

Cucurbite.

The manufacture of the alchemical gold which is the Dew of Immortality consists of a peculiar operation having several phases. Through the stimulus of warmth and spiritual fire to the Athanor there should be a transfer, an ascent of the Serpent from that instrument into the Cucurbite, used as a retort. The alchemical marriage or the mingling of the two streams of force in the retort causes at once the chemical corruption of the Serpent in the menstruum of the Gluten, this being the *solvé* part of the general alchemical formula of *solvé et coagula*. Hard upon the corruption of the Serpent and his death, arises the resplendent Phoenix which, as a talisman, should be charged by means of a continuous invocation of the spiritual principle conforming to the work in hand. The conclusion of the Mass consists in either the consumption of the trans-substantiated elements, which is the Amrita, or the anointing and consecration of a special talisman.

Prior to proceeding further with the analysis of aspects of this operation, I should like to place before the reader a quotation wherein this Mass is repeated at some length, using the conventional nomenclature of alchemy. "I am a goddess for beauty and extraction famous, born out of our proper sea which compasseth the whole earth and is ever restless. Out of my breasts I pour forth milk and blood; boil these two till they are turned into silver and gold. O most excellent subject, out of which all things are generated, though at first sight thou art poison, adorned with the name of the Flying Eagle . . . Thy parents are the Sun and Moon; in thee there is water and wine, gold also and silver upon earth, that mortal man may rejoice . . . But consider, O man, what things God bestows upon thee by this means. Torture the Eagle till she weeps and the Lion be weakened and bleed to death. The blood of this Lion incorporated with the tears of the Eagle is the treasure of the earth." This, without doubt, is also in explanation of the figure reproduced by Franz Hartman.

By some authorities, it is roughly estimated that from the preliminary Invocation, with the binding of the force in the elements, to the act of partaking the communion itself from the consecrated Chalice, the operation should not take less than an hour. Sometimes, indeed, a much longer period is required, especially if it is required that the charging of the talisman be complete and thorough. Great care is required to prevent the unguarded loss of the elements. There is the possibility of actual leakage or an overflowing from the Cucurbite, and the assimilation or evaporation of the corrupted elements within that instrument is also an accident greatly to be deplored.

It cannot be stressed too strongly or too frequently that if the elements are not consecrated aright; or in the first place if the invoked force does not properly impinge upon or is insecurely bound within the elements, the whole operation may be nullified. And it may easily degenerate to the lowest depths, resulting in the creation of a Qliphotic horror to exist like a vampire upon the unnaturally sensitive and those who are inclinded to hysteria and obsession. If the elixir be properly distilled, serving as the medium of the invoked spirit, then the Heavens are opened, and the Gates swing back for the Theurgist, and the treasures of the earth are laid at his feet. "If you discover it be silent and keep it sacred. Trust to nobody but to God."

The problem of the link to connect the magical operation with the desired result should be considered in all its numerous aspects. If the Operation is one actually requiring an exterior talisman for the visible production of its effect, a suitable seal should be constructed in metal, wax, or on parchment. It may be consecrated and anointed with the elixir which has been created through the channels of the Hermetic Work. Those seals and talismans described in the *Key of Solomon the King* and *The Magus* are for the purpose quite suitable.

Should it be that the operation proposed by the Theurgist is one pertaining to the qualities of Jupiter, a

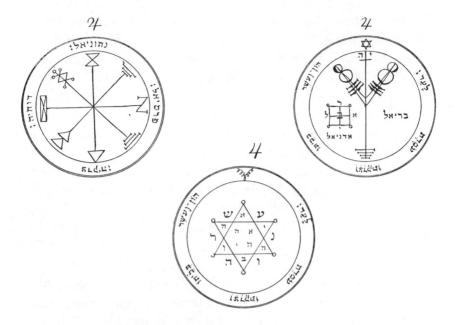

suitable pantacle should be prepared before the Operation. During the manufacture of the Elixir, the God-Mask of Maat should be assumed, and a conjuration of the required angel or intelligence recited. Upon the completion of the Mass a minute quantity of the supernal dew should be placed on the sigil or talisman of Jupiter thus charging it with an insuperable force for the production of the desired results. Variations of this procedure will probably occur with practice.

No question of a link enters into a ceremony conducted for an end wherein the Circle and the Triangle, so to speak, or the demon and the exorcist, occupy the same plane. That is, when the Theurgist works solely upon his own consciousness without reference to any exterior effect. The Mass of the Holy Ghost, in such a case, is automatically climaxed by the consumption of the charged elements, the invoked force incarnating with the Magician as a matter of course. It is in this type of operation, I think, that the Mass of the Holy Ghost generates the greatest amount of force and ascends to the highest level of efficiency.

Even for ordinary operations, the great advantage of this method is that ceremonial may be dispensed with almost altogether. The Magician quite easily can perform the banishing ritual on the Astral, and the invocations may be silently recited so that no Magic of a ceremonial nature may be perceived by the profane. In the instance of operations, however, where the result desired exists on another plane or exterior to the consciousness of the Magician, effects do not always seem to follow with the same infallibility and sequence as they do in subjective workings.

The perusal of private records kept by Magicians who have utilized this magical engine tend to show that it is best employed for works within the consciousness of the Magician. It is in these matters that the Mass of the Holy Ghost is the most puissant and efficacious. For the development of the Magical Will, the enhancement of the Imagination, and the Invocation both of Adonai and the Universal Gods to indwell the consecrated temple of the Holy Ghost, a better or more suitable method could hardly be devised. No expenditure of vital energy is involved, for any energy so utilized in the operation returns at the end to the Magician enhanced and enriched with the birth of the golden Phoenix, the symbol of resurrection and rebirth.

The supreme power operating in this technique is *love*. Trite though it may seem, hackneyed though the word itself has become, it must be reiterated that love is the motivating power; a love force held always in leash by the *Will* and controlled by the *Soul*. The destructive power of the Sword and all that the Sword implies, the dispersive character of the Dagger or any of the other elemental weapons, has no place herein. This method therefore commends itself as being of the very highest. Since it does partake of love, it is of the stuff and essence of life itself.

In operation, this Mass is extraordinarily simple. Indeed, one Magus has observed that it is no more compli-

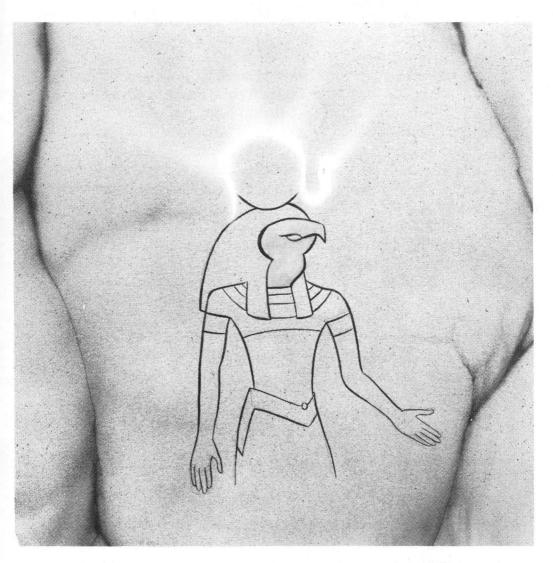

Ra

cated than the riding of a bicycle; that is to say, when once certain preliminaries and training have been encompassed. More than anything else it requires a peculiarly potent and detached Will, arguing of course previous discipline, and a mind which has been trained to concentration for long periods of time. One of the peculiarities of this technique is that unless one is exceptionally wary and alert from the beginning, it is an easy matter for the Magician to lose control of his alchemical instruments, and thus spoil the entire operation. Joy in the mere technical performance of the Mass to the exclusion of proper magical work constitutes the great and supreme danger. On the other hand, because this element of delight and joy does enter into it, this technique commands excellence over all others. The mind must be trained to concentrate under all circumstances. As a preliminary to magical practice of this kind, the technique of Yoga is a tremendous advantage. One may even state that for true success in all Magic, a thorough grounding in Yoga technique is an absolute essential.

A further observation may not be out of place. On the surface and at first sight it may appear that between this type of magical operation, so hesitatingly described, and the usual ceremonial working there exists a wide gap. It is true that the Mass of the Holy Ghost is an advance on the cumbrous and slow working of ceremonial, even although the latter is an essential at the commencement of magical training. This method is considerably more direct and to the point, and because of the peculiar class of energies which it brings to bear upon Nature, its effects are exceedingly more powerful and far-reaching than those of ceremonial alone. Nevertheless, although subsisting as two distinct classes of work, they can with great advantage be combined and used one in conjunction with the other.

The general consensus of opinion of the alchemical authorities, by whom this method was esteemed, was that lofty as it was, its results could not be encompassed without prayer. Without sincere prayer nothing permanent or divine could be accomplished. Hence, while the operation of the Mass is in progress, and the fire in the Athanor becomes more intense, an enthusiastic invocation, either astral or audible, should be recited. It should be in the nature of a short mantram appropriate to the nature and type of working, rhythmical in composition. The operation as a whole could be preceded by a more general invocation to legitimize the work. As the astral work of creation proceeds, the rhythmical mantram will help to formulate and vivify the moulds caused by Will and Imagination, attracting the spiritual force desired. Then, when the Serpent is transferred from the Athanor and the alchemical corruption commences in the Gluten of the White Eagle, the cucurbite will be the receptacle of a new substance, living and dynamic, bearing the indelible impress of the invocations that will have endowed its plasticity and potentiality with an overwhelming impetus in a given direction. It will follow that with the partaking of this substance which is the philosophical Mercury, impregnated with an intelligence of dynamic spiritual energy capable of producing within the confines of its sphere the desired change, complete and satisfactory fulfillment climaxes the aspiration of the Magician.

Conducted within a properly consecrated Circle, after a thorough banishing, followed by a mighty conjuration of the divine force, and the assumption of the appropriate God-form, the ceremony may prove of incomparable power to open wide the Gates of the Heavens. Using solely the Cup and the Wand as elemental weapons, together with the mantram or the specialized rhythmic invocation, the Mass can seldom fail of effect. This union of two different magical weapons, far apart though they may have appeared in the first instance, enhance the potency of each, since they combine in a single operation the finest aspects and the greatest advantages of both.

Appendix B: Rite of the Naked Fire

FIRST PUBLISHED 15 years ago in India, by Shri Mahendranath of Gujarat, this superb ritual has multiple flexibility. The ritual may be used by groups, couples or individuals as a consciousness altering preliminary to solitary Kriya practice of right hand Tantra or as preparation by a couple for left hand (Vama Marg) sexual experiences.

David Ramsdale and Ellen Dorfman in their excellent book, *Sexual Energy Ecstasy,* point out that the word "rite" and "right" are semantic cousins. The truth of ritual significance may be revealed at a deeper level when we realize that the English word "ritual" (hence "rite") etymologically derives from the Sanskrit prefix *ri,* "to flow with or away with." Indeed, the value of a sexual ritual or ceremony becomes even more evident when we know that the etymological root of "ceremony" is also Sanskrit—literally *karmamony,* i.e. the doctrine that every action has a consequence and therefore the value of careful and correct ceremony is

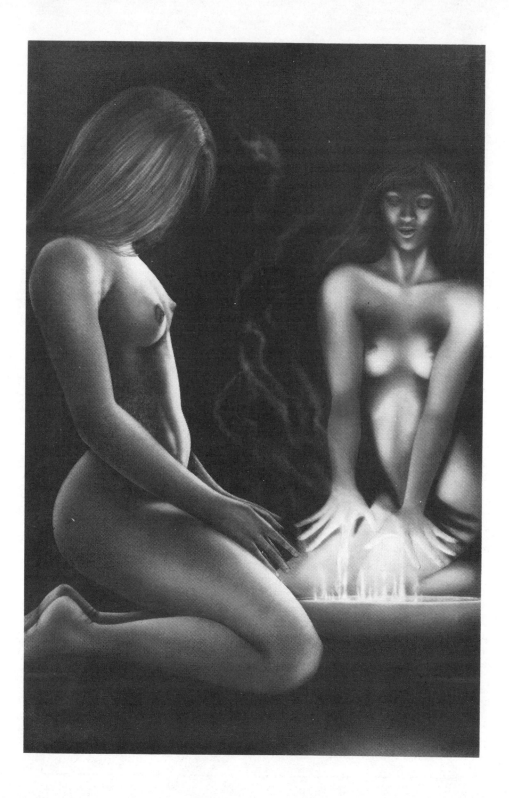

to ensure the consequences of the activity are benign.

That which follows is Shri Mahendranath's commentary and translation.

Rite of the Naked Fire

By Shri Mahendranath the Avadhuta:
Gujarat

Most sects of Sannyasins, of Tantric or Yoga traditions, associated with Shiva, Shiva-Shakti, or the Mother Goddess observe the custom, the origin of which is lost in antiquity, of keeping a sacred fire burning in any place where they stay for a period. This fire is lit in a circular *Dhunee* made of mud and stones, and it's lighting is initiated with some ritual. These cults do not worship fire, but the *Dhunee*, once lit, is regarded as sacred, and the ashes are used to smear and mark the body, and also are given to visitors for the same purpose.

If the rite is performed in a building or home, a metal or earthenware bowl can be used. The fire can be very small and the flames can be fed with *Ghee* or vegetable oils. Mineral oil, paper or chemicals must not be used. Once the rite is completed the Sadhus leave it to smoulder, and add wood or dried cow-dung as necessary. If performed in a home, or as a private ceremony, it need not be kept burning longer than the actual need. This rite of the Naked Fire is the one used by the Adi-Nath Sect of Nathas. The words, originally Sanskrit, are here rendered in English. Only the Mantras of the invocation must be retained in their original form. OM prefaces all Manatras, and it is put there to imply that whatever is expressed in the Mantra, it is still only OM.

Attention should be paid to the wording of the rite, if it is not to become only a worthless ritual. Each verse expresses basic Upanishad teachings, and they can expand one's awareness. Most Sannyasin sects have a strict tradition that they must be naked when meditating, performing the fire rite, and, as sometimes done by new young Sadhus, when doing *Puja* or worship. A rite of this kind is an ideal opening for group meditation, or for the practice and teaching of Yoga. In such circumstances one person should light and tend the fire, while another chants the Mantras and text.

Fire rites differ considerably among different sects and Guru schools. This rite of the Naked Fire, although modern in its presentation, preserves that Golden Thread which runs through Hindu Paganism, and it expresses most of all the Teachings of Sri Dattatreya and the Adi-Nathas. Fire rites in non-Aryan Paganism are not exclusive to Sadhus, and may be performed by householders and students.

THE INVOCATION

OM NAMAH SHIVAYA!
OM NAMAH SHIVAYA!   (Salutation to Lord Shiva)
OM NAMAH SHIVAYA!

HARA HARA MAHADEVA,   (Hara is the Great God,
   SHIVA-SHAMBU,   Shiva Shambu, Lord of
KASHI VISHWANATHA   the world, residing at Kashi
   GANGA!   on the Ganges)

OM GURUR BRAHMA,   (The Guru is Brahma, the
   GURUR VISHNU,   Guru is Vishnu,
   GURU DEVA MAHESH-   The Guru is also
      WARA;   Shiva Maheshwara
   GURUS SHAKSHAT   The Guru is the
      PARAMBRAHMAN,   Absolute
   TASMAI SHRI GURUVE   Salutations to the
      NAMAH!   Guru)

THE ORATION

"One fire, One God, One world, One people;
Ignorance transforms the One into many:
Homage and Salutations to the Naked Fire!

"As fire burns we destroy delusion and bondage,
Leaving only the white ash of Liberation.
Homage and Salutations to the Naked Fire!

"Let the fire destroy the drag of the senses,
Pulling us hither and thither in bondage;
Homage and Salutations to the Naked Fire!

"In the Naked Fire the mind regenerated,
Fit to attain the vision of Reality.
Homage and Salutations to the Naked Fire!

"As burning releases the fire from the fuel,
May mankind be released from bondage.
Homage and Salutations to the Naked Fire!

"Let the fire burn all Karmas and their power,
Releasing us to attain equipoise and Liberation.
Homage and Salutations to the Naked Fire!

"The flame in the fire is the symbol of Wisdom;
As Naked Fire let the inner Consciousness glow.
Homage and Salutations to the Naked Fire!

"Realisation of the Self is Immortality
And the Supreme Attainment is spontaneous.
Homage and Salutations to the Naked Fire!

"Thoughtless, the fire burns without intention;
In Samadhi we attain that state of Bliss.
Homage and Salutations to the Naked Fire!

"Like as the *Dhunee* is the symbol of Shakti,
The flame is the *Lingam* of Lord Shiva.
Homage and Salutations to the Naked Fire!

"As above, so below. Fuel transforms to ash;
All the worlds in the Universe turn to dust.
Homage and Salutations to the Naked Fire!

"As fire is inherent in the fuel,
So the Soul is inherent in the body.
Homage and Salutations to the Sacred Fire!

"In the fires of *Samsara,* painfully burning;
May the Grace of the Absolute descend on us.
Homage and Salutations to the Sacred Fire!

As fire takes the form of the fuel it consumes,
The Immortal Soul takes the form of the body.
Homage and Salutations to the Sacred Fire!

As flame passes on to other pieces of wood,
So the Soul passes on from body to body.
Homage and Salutations to the Sacred Fire!

"Drink though the Nectar of Immortality;
Thou art the Naked Fire of Eternity.
Homage and Salutations to the Naked Fire!

In the fire of frustration, Wisdom is born,
From the womb of a jackal, a tiger is born,
From the fire of Wisdom, dispassion is born,
From all cast aside, Liberation is born.
Then one has done all that which needs be done,
As Naked Fire then shine as mortals all.
Homage and Salutations to the Naked Fire!"

OM NAMAH SHIVAYA!
OM NAMAH SHIVAYA!
OM NAMAH SHIVAYA!
OM SHANTI SHANTI SHANTI!

A Note on the Khajuraho Photography

The magnificent photographs taken by Melissa Jade, a microbiologist, are part of a large collection involving three months' research we undertook in Khajuraho, Madhya Pradesh state, Central India, 1984.

They are only a small sample of what has become one of the largest collections outside India. I have utilized them in this second edition to illustrate Indian concepts of feminine pulchritude, particularly the erotic mode, as the supreme concept of the aesthetic experience.

It must be emphasized, contrary to both popular and academic opinion, that the erotic art of Khajuraho has nothing to do with Tantra. This is true despite the existence of a Shakti cult as evidenced by the Chausath-yogini temple, probably built in the late 900's A.D.

The multitude of exquisite figures adorning the temples at Khajuraho, concentrated on the outside but by no means absent from the interiors, represent art, pure and simple. A thousand years ago the ultimate flowering of Indian erotic sculpture took place under the benevolent patronage of the Chandella dynasty. The evidence for this we will present in a future book and thesis.

Jonn Mumford
Melissa Jade
Sydney, Australia, 1985

Research Bibliography

CHAPTER ONE: *The Sorcery of Love*

Ahmed, Rollo. *The Black Art.* London: John Lang Ltd., 1936.

Crowley, A. *Magick in Theory and Practice.* Paris: Lecram Press, 1929.

Dane, Victor. *The Gateway to Prosperity.* London: Master Key Co., 1937.

Regardie, Israel. *The Tree of Life.* London: Rider and Co., 1932.

Waite, A.E. *The Holy Kabbalah.* London: Williams and Norgate, 1929.

CHAPTER TWO: *Tantra*

Bharati, Swami Agehananda. *The Ochre Robe.* London: George Allen and Unwin Ltd., 1961.

Bharati, Swami Agehananda. *The Tantric Tradition.* London: Rider and Company, 1965.

Eliade, Mircea. *Yoga: Immortality and Freedom.* New York, N.Y., U.S.A.: Bollingen Foundation Inc., 1958.

Huard, Pierre and Ming Wong. *Chinese Medicine.* London: World University Library, 1968.

Zimmer, H. *Philosophies of India.* New York: Meridian Books, Inc., 1958.

CHAPTER THREE: *Psycho-Sexual Power*

Brecher, Ruth and Edward. *An Analysis of Human Sexual Response.* London: Panther Books, 1968.

Crowley, Aleister. *Yoga.* Dallas, Texas: Sangreal Foundation, 1969.

Saraswati, Swami Satyananda. *Asana, Pranayama, Mudra, Bandha.* Monghyr, India: Bihar School of Yoga, 1973.

_____. *Dynamics of Yoga,* Monghyr, India: Bihar School of Yoga, 1966.

CHAPTER FOUR: *Asanas of Love*

Avalon, Arthur. *The Serpent Power.* Madras, India: Ganesh and Co., 1953.

Culling, Louis T. *The Complete Magick Curriculum of the Secret Order G∴B∴G∴.* St. Paul, Minnesota: Llewellyn, 1970.

Ishihara, Akira and Howards-Levy. *The Tao of Sex.* New York: Harper and Row, 1970.

Luk, Charles. *Taoist Yoga, Alchemy and Immortality.* London: Rider and Company, 1970.

Rama, S. *Ananga Ranga.* Amritsan: Brijmohan and Co., Publishers, 1933.

Rele, V.G. *The Mysterious Kundalini.* D.B. Taraporevala Sons and Co., 1931.

_____ . *The Vedic Gods as Figures of Biology.* D.B. Taraporevala Sons and Co., 1931.

Vatsyayana. *Kama Sutra.* New York: Lancer Books, 1964.

CHAPTER FIVE: *A Tantric Synopic Commentary on the Shat Chakras*

Avalon, Arthur. *The Serpent Power.* Madras, India: Ganesh and Co., 1953.

Saraswati, Swami Satyananda. *Asana, Pranayama, Mudra, Bandha.* Monghyr, India: Bihar School of Yoga, 1973.

CHAPTER SIX: *Sexual Terminology: Semantics of the Inner Life*

Bhandarkar, Sri Ramkrishna Gopal. *First Book of Sanskrit.* Bombay: Karnatak Publishing House, 1957.

Pocket Oxford Dictionary of Current English, The. Clarendon Press, 1955.

Scott, George Ryley. *Phallic Worship.* London: Panther Books, 1970.

Skeat, Rev. Walter W. *A Concise Etymological Dictionary of the English Language.* New York: Capricorn Books, 1963.

Tantra. Arts Council of Great Britain Publications, 1972.

Webster's Complete English Dictionary. George Bell and Sons, 1886.

Webster Universal Dictionary. Routledge and Kegan Paul Ltd., 1968.

Wedeck, Harry E., *Dictionary of Aphrodisiacs.* New York: The Citadel Press, 1962.

CHAPTER SEVEN: *Eros and Thantos*

A.A. Brill. *Lectures on Psychoanalytic Psychiatry.* New York: Vintage Books, 1955.

Colville, Costello and Rouke. *Abnormal Psychology.* New York, N.Y.: Barnes and Noble Inc., 1960.

Freud, Sigmund. *A General Introduction to Psychoanalysis.* New York: Garden City Publishing Co., 1938.

Smith, Sir Sydney and Frederick Smith Fiddes. *Forensic Medicine.* London: J.&A. Churchill Ltd., 1955.

Walton, A.H. *Aphrodisiacs.* Westport, Conn., U.S.A.: Associated Booksellers, 1958.

CHAPTER EIGHT: *Tantra, Modern Witchcraft and Psychedelic Drugs*

Huxley, Aldous. *Visionary Experience.* Copenhagen: Proceedings of the XIV International Congress of Applied Psychology, Vol. 4, August 13-19.

King, Francis. *Sexuality, Magic and Perversion.* London: New English Library of Occult Series, 1972.

Saraswati, Swami Satyananda. *Tantra-Yoga Panorama.* Rajanandgaon M.P. India: International Yoga Fellowship Movement, 1972.

_____.*Tantra of Kundalini Yoga.* Monghyr, India: Bihar School of Yoga, 1973.

Walker, Benjamin. *Sex and the Supernatural.* London: Macdonald Unit 75, 1970.

STAY IN TOUCH

On the following pages you will find listed, with their current prices, some of the books now available on related subjects. Your book dealer stocks most of these and will stock new titles in the Llewellyn series as they become available. We urge your patronage.

To obtain our full catalog, to keep informed about new titles as they are released and to benefit from informative articles and helpful news, you are invited to write for our bimonthly news magazine/catalog, *Llewellyn's New Worlds of Mind and Spirit*. A sample copy is free, and it will continue coming to you at no cost as long as you are an active mail customer. Or you may subscribe for just $7.00 in the U.S.A. and Canada ($20.00 overseas, first class mail). Many bookstores also have *New Worlds* available to their customers. Ask for it.

Stay in touch! In *New Worlds'* pages you will find news and features about new books, tapes and services, announcements of meetings and seminars, articles helpful to our readers, news of authors, products and services, special money-making opportunities, and much more.

Llewellyn's New Worlds of Mind and Spirit
P.O. Box 64383-494, St. Paul, MN 55164-0383, U.S.A.
* * *

TO ORDER BOOKS AND TAPES

If your book dealer does not have the books described on the following pages readily available, you may order them directly from the publisher by sending full price in U.S. funds, plus $3.00 for postage and handling for orders *under* $10.00; $4.00 for orders *over* $10.00. There are no postage and handling charges for orders over $50.00. Postage and handling rates are subject to change. UPS Delivery: We ship UPS whenever possible. Delivery guaranteed. Provide your street address as UPS does not deliver to P.O. Boxes. UPS to Canada requires a $50.00 minimum order. Allow 4-6 weeks for delivery. Orders outside the U.S.A. and Canada: Airmail—add retail price of book; add $5.00 for each non-book item (tapes, etc.); add $1.00 per item for surface mail.

FOR GROUP STUDY AND PURCHASE

Because there is a great deal of interest in group discussion and study of the subject matter of this book, we feel that we should encourage the adoption and use of this particular book by such groups by offering a special quantity price to group leaders or agents.

Our special quantity price for a minimum order of five copies of *Ecstasy Through Tantra* is $38.85 cash-with-order. This price includes postage and handling within the United States. Minnesota residents must add 6.5% sales tax. For additional quantities, please order in multiples of five. For Canadian and foreign orders, add postage and handling charges as above. Credit card (VISA, MasterCard, American Express) orders are accepted. Charge card orders only ($15.00 minimum order) may be phoned in free within the U.S.A. or Canada by dialing 1-800-THE-MOON. For customer service, call 1-612-291-1970. Mail orders to:

LLEWELLYN PUBLICATIONS
P.O. Box 64383-494, St. Paul, MN 55164-0383, U.S.A.

SEX MAGICK
by Louis T. Culling

In sexual union there is a uniting of magnetic and electric currents to create a field of energy that extends both inward and outward to contact the infinite Intelligence and the personal unconscious. In perfecting this union lies Magick, for we gain insight and extend our personal power by becoming a channel to the powers of the universe.

In *Sex Magick* the long hidden secrets and principles of sex magick are revealed with examples that enable one to turn sexual union into a valid tool for mystical ecstasy and self-transcendence.

This is *not* the magic of sex; Sex Magick is using sex as a potent vehicle for magical attainment. Its purpose is to accomplish the mystical union of normal consciousness with the highest consciousness. It embraces a healthy psychological view of man, allowing him to grow and create without restriction. Sex Magick is unsurpassed for achieving the highest physical and spiritual ecstasies.
0-87542-110-5, 148 pages, 5¼ x 8, softcover.   **$6.95**

THE GOLDEN DAWN
by Israel Regardie

The Original Account of the Teachings, Rites and Ceremonies of the Hermetic Order of the Golden Dawn as revealed by Israel Regardie, with further revision, expansion, and additional notes by Israel Regardie, Cris Monnastre, and others. Originally published in four volumes of some 1200 pages, this 5th Edition has been entirely reset in modern type, in half the pages (while retaining the original pagination in marginal notation for reference) for greater ease and use.

Corrections of typographical errors in the original edition have been made, with further revision and additional text and notes by actual practitioners of the Golden Dawn system, with an Introduction by the only student ever accepted for personal training by Regardie.

Also included are Initiation Ceremonies, rituals for consecration and invocation, methods of magical working based on the Enochian Tablets, studies in the Tarot, and the system of Qabalistic Correspondences that unite religions and magical traditions into a comprehensive whole.

This volume is designed as a study and practice curriculum suited to both group and private practice. Meditation upon, and following with the Active Imagination, the Initiation Ceremonies is fully experiential without need of participation in group or lodge.
0-87542-663-8, 744 pages, 6 x 9, illus.   **$19.95**

A GARDEN OF POMEGRANATES
by Israel Regardie
What is the Tree of Life? It's the ground plan of the Qabalistic system—a set of symbols used since ancient times to study the Universe. The Tree of Life is a geometrical arrangement of ten sephiroth, or spheres, each of which is associated with a different archetypal idea, and 22 paths which connect the spheres.

This system of primal correspondences has been found the most efficient plan ever devised to classify and organize the characteristics of the self. Israel Regardie has written one of the best and most lucid introductions to the Qabalah.

A Garden of Pomegranates combines Regardie's own studies with his notes on the works of Aleister Crowley, A. E. Waite, Eliphas Levi and D. H. Lawrence. No longer is the wisdom of the Qabalah to be held secret! The needs of today place the burden of growth upon each and every person— each has to undertake the Path as his or her own responsibility, but every help is given in the most ancient and yet most modern teaching here known to humankind.

0-87542-690-5,160 pgs., 5-1/4 x 8, softcover **$8.95**

THE MIDDLE PILLAR
by Israel Regardie
Between the two outer pillars of the Qabalistic Tree of Life, the extremes of Mercy and Severity, stands THE MIDDLE PILLAR, signifying one who has achieved equilibrium in his or her own self.

Integration of the human personality is vital to the continuance of creative life. Without it, man lives as an outsider to his own true self. By combining Magic and Psychology in the Middle Pillar Ritual/Exercise (a magical meditation technique),we bring into balance the opposing elements of the psyche while yet holding within their essence and allowing full expression of man's entire being.

In this book, and with this practice, you will learn to: understand the psyche through its correspondences on the Tree of Life; expand self-awareness, thereby intensifying the inner growth process; activate creative and intuitive potentials; understand the individual thought patterns which control every facet of personal behavior; regain the sense of balance and peace of mind—the equilibrium that everyone needs for physical and psychic health.

0-87542-658-1, 176 pgs., 5-1/4 x 8, softcover **$8.95**

MODERN MAGICK
by Don Kraig
Modern Magick is the most comprehensive step-by-step introduction to the art of ceremonial magic ever offered. The eleven lessons in this book will guide you from the easiest of rituals and the construction of your magickal tools through the highest forms of magick: designing your own rituals and doing pathworking. Along the way you will learn the secrets of the Kabbalah in a clear and easy-to-understand manner. You will also discover the true secrets of invocation (channeling) and evocation, and the missing information that will finally make the ancient *grimoires*, such as the **Keys of Solomon**, not only comprehensible, but usable. *Modern Magick* is designed so anyone can use it, and is the perfect guidebook for students and classes. It will also help to round out the knowledge of long-time practitioners of the magickal arts.

0-87542-324-8, 608 pgs., 6 x 9, illus., softcover **$14.95**

MYSTERIA MAGICA
by Denning and Phillips

For years, Denning and Phillips headed the international occult Order Aurum Solis. In this book they present the magickal system of the order so that you can use it. Here you will find rituals for banishing and invoking plus instructions for proper posture and breathing. You will learn astral projection, rising on the planes, and the magickal works that should be undertaken through astral projection. You will learn the basic principle of ceremonies and how to make sigils and talismans. You will learn practical Enochian magick plus how to create, consecrate and use your magickal tools such as the magickal sword, wand and cup. You will also learn the advanced arts of sphere-working and evocation to visible appearance.

Filled with illustrations, this book is an expanded version of the previous edition. It is now complete in itself and can be the basis of an entire magickal system. You can use the information alone or as the source book for a group. It is volume 3 of *The Magical Philosophy*, the other two books being *The Sword and The Serpent* and *The Foundations of High Magick*. If you want to learn how to do real magick, this is the place you should start.

0-87542-196-2, 480 pgs., 6 x 9, illus., softcover $15.00

WHEELS OF LIFE: A User's Guide to the Chakra System
by Anodea Judith

An instruction manual for owning and operating the inner gears that run the machinery of our lives. Written in a practical, down-to-earth style, this fully-illustrated book will take the reader on a journey through aspects of consciousness, from the bodily instincts of survival to the processing of deep thoughts.

Discover this ancient metaphysical system under the new light of popular Western metaphors—quantum physics, elemental magick, Kabbalah, physical exercises, poetic meditations, and visionary art. Learn how to open these centers in yourself, and see how the chakras shed light on the present world crises we face today. And learn what you can do about it!

This book will be a vital resource for: Magicians, Witches, Pagans, Mystics, Yoga Practitioners, Martial Arts people, Psychologists, Medical people, and all those who are concerned with holistic growth techniques.

The modern picture of the Chakras was introduced to the West largely in the context of Hatha and Kundalini Yoga and through the Theosophical writings of Leadbeater and Besant. But the Chakra system is equally innate to Western Magick: all psychic development, spiritual growth, and practical attainment is fully dependent upon the opening of the Chakras!

0-87542-320-5, 544 pgs., 6 x 9, illus., softcover $12.95

THE LLEWELLYN ANNUALS

Llewellyn's MOON SIGN BOOK: Approximately 400 pages of valuable information on gardening, fishing, weather, stock market forecasts, personal horoscopes, good planting dates, and general instructions for finding the best date to do just about anything! Article by prominent forecasters and writers in the fields of gardening, astrology, politics, economics and cycles. This special almanac, different from any other, has been published annually since 1906. It's fun, informative and has been a great help to millions in their daily planning.　　**State year $4.95**

Llewellyn's SUN SIGN BOOK: Your personal horoscope for the entire year! All 12 signs are included in one handy book. Also included are forecasts, special feature articles, and an action guide for each sign. Monthly horoscopes are written by Gloria Star, author of *Optimum Child*, for your personal Sun Sign and there are articles on a variety of subjects written by well-known astrologers from around the country. Much more than just a horoscope guide! Entertaining and fun the year around.　　**State year $4.95**

Llewellyn's DAILY PLANETARY GUIDE and ASTROLOGER'S DATEBOOK: Includes all of the major daily aspects plus their exact times in Eastern and Pacific time zones, lunar phases, signs and voids plus their times, planetary motion, a monthly ephemeris, sunrise and sunset tables, special articles on the planets, signs, aspects, a business guide, planetary hours, rulerships, and much more. Large 5.25 x 8 format for more writing space, spiral bound to lay flat, address and phone listings, time zone conversion chart and blank horoscope chart.　　**State year $6.95**

Llewellyn's ASTROLOGICAL CALENDAR: Large wall calendar of 48 pages. Beautiful full color cover and full color inside. Includes special feature articles by famous astrologers, and complete introductory information on astrology. It also contains a Lunar Gardening Guide, celestial phenomena, a blank horoscope chart, and monthly date pages which include aspects, Moon phases, signs and voids, planetary motion, an ephemeris, personal forecasts, lucky dates, planting and fishing dates, and more. 10 x 13 size. Set in Central time, with fold-down conversion table for other time zones worldwide.　　**State year $9.95**

PRACTICAL SIGIL MAGIC
by Frater U∴D∴
This powerful magical system is right for anyone who has the desire to change his/her life! Frater U D shows you how to create personal sigils (signs) using your unconscious. Artistic skill is not a necessity in drawing sigils, but honest, straightforward, precise intentions are. Based on Austin Osman Spare's theory of sigils and the Alphabet of Desire, *Practical Sigil Magic* explores the background of this magical practice as well as specific methods, such as the word method with its *sentence of desire*. The pictorial and mantrical spell methods are also explained with many illustrations. The last chapter is devoted solely to creating sigils from planetary cameas.

Once you've created your sigil, you'll learn how to internalize or activate it, finally banishing it from your consciousness as it works imperceptibly in the outer world. Let Frater U D , a leading magician of Germany, take you on this magical journey to the center of your dreams.
0-87542-774-X, 166 pgs., 5¼ x 8, illus., softcover   **$8.95**